UNDERSTANDING BABIES

UNDERSTANDING BABIES

How engaging with your baby's movement
development helps build a loving relationship

ANIA WITKOWSKA

pinter
&
martin

Understanding Babies: How engaging with your baby's movement development helps build a loving relationship

First published by Pinter & Martin Ltd 2021

ISBN 978-1-78066-680-8

Editor: Susan Last
Index: Helen Bilton

British Library Cataloguing-in-Publication Data
A catalogue record for this book is available from the British Library

Printed by TJ Books Limited, Padstow, Cornwall

This book has been printed on paper that is sourced and harvested from sustainable forests and is FSC accredited

Pinter & Martin Ltd
6 Effra Parade
London SW2 1PS

www.pinterandmartin.com

CONTENTS

PUBLISHER'S NOTE

Ania Witkowska, mother of three, somatic movement therapist and educator, died in 2019 at the age of 56. This book, which she was completing in the weeks before she died, is derived from over 20 years' experience working with parents and babies in workshops, classes and one-to-one therapeutic situations. It is her legacy to parents and new babies everywhere.

ABOUT THE AUTHOR

Ania Witkowska led movement development programmes for 'babies, children and their grown-ups' in Manchester based on her training in community art practice, interest in contemporary dance, and studies in somatics, integrative bodywork and movement therapy. When she moved to Germany with her husband and three children in 2006 she developed this further, working as a movement therapist and educator in Berlin, Vilnius and Moscow until her death in 2019. Her delight in fostering responsive parenting through movement permeated every aspect of her work.

AUTHOR'S NOTE

The information in this book is based on my training as a somatic movement educator and therapist as well as my professional and personal experience as a mother of three. It's a journey that started with the birth of my first child in 1995 and grew out of my frustration at the lack of quality information about how she was developing. The choice was to either 'do what I was told' by an expert, or to relax and 'learn from my baby'. I have to admit I have never been one to do what I was told without a whole lot of questions, so I was drawn to the latter option. But when I looked at the curled-up bundle in my arms I didn't know where to start: it was hard to know how to interpret what I saw. Was she arching her back because she had tummy ache, or did she simply enjoy a stretch? Did sucking her hands indicate hunger or something else? I spent my time with my baby in a state of mild anxiety and bewilderment. My emotions would alternate between the weight of responsibility and the lightness of total love. Increasingly tired, I also often felt lonely and bored and then of course guilty for being anything less than ecstatic about parenthood.

Once the first shock had worn off and my brain started to rebalance I turned to what I knew best: movement. My work as a community dance practitioner was with young children, and I had recently discovered the work of Bonnie Bainbridge Cohen, the originator of Body Mind Centering®. She talked about movement milestones as part of a larger developmental movement sequence, which underpins our ability to focus, study and learn. I had started to introduce these elements into my dance sessions and teachers were noticing some positive changes. Now, with a small baby living with me and experiencing the sequence, I could delve deeper. In the mid-1990s Body Mind Centering® was little known outside the world of dance and performance. Indeed, before Wikipedia and laptops the world was a very different place. Niche information was hard to come by living in Manchester. I persuaded a friend going to New York to bring me back a copy of *Sensing, Feeling, and Action*, a book of Bonnie's writings. I started to study on my own, with my daughter and later my young son beside me on the floor.

As I tried out the movements with them I was able to gain insight into the way my babies might be feeling, how much effort was needed and what practical elements would give them support. I noticed how easy it was to get in the way of their efforts, without realising what you were doing. With their two very different personalities I was more aware of how each needed different things from me.

As my children grew older I was able to pursue my studies formally. I started the new century by attending a short course called 'Engaging the Whole Child' at the School for Body Mind Centering® in the USA, and in 2003 began diploma studies at Linda Hartley's

Institute for Integrative Bodywork and Movement Therapy. Linda's programme included somatic and developmental psychology, as well as an in-depth study of infant movement development. We studied the work of psychologists and psychotherapists like Daniel Stern, Peter Levine, Ruella Frank and Frances La Barre, and I saw how movement and touch expressed and established our relationship with our children.

My move to Berlin in 2006 with my now-larger family (my third child was born in 2004) allowed me to grow my work. I developed the Understanding Babies Parent Education programme and ran classes and workshops. In sessions parents looked at the world from the babies' perspectives: they physically explored what their babies did, mirroring their babies on the floor. They observed how each baby's individuality shone through the general themes they were learning. I offered ideas for games and play activities to try, and basic principles from my dance background that made them feel more confident in handling and playing with their babies. By observing and following the babies' lead, parents could see how each baby set their own learning agenda, and how they could support rather than hinder that process. We moved, played and had a lot of fun!

Before long I became aware that the work was also benefiting the parents. By revisiting the developmental movement sequence parents were building up their ability to listen and be aware of their own bodies, and this was deeply resourcing them. I watched people become more comfortable, less anxious and better able to trust and follow their instincts. And the babies responded: they were calmer and better able to modulate their emotions. The connection between parent and child grew stronger. A subtle difference in the way the babies were being seen became evident. We observed the babies with respect, not judging, nor pushing them towards achievements. We enjoyed their independent learning and joined in to support them appropriately when they told us they needed our help. It was clear that by attending to movement and touch the work had also nourished that vital relationship between parent and baby.

I hope this book enriches and nourishes your parenting journey.

What is 'somatics' and what is somatic movement education?

Think about the way you sense your body differently barefoot in the morning grass, or in shoes on the street; the feeling you encounter in a large open space or deep in the woods, the image that pops into your mind when observing a child absorbed in play: these are all somatic moments. Your lived experience, how you feel within yourself, how you sense, and are touched by, the moving world around you is your somatic perspective. So we might say that a somatic experience is a fully lived experience, the moments when you are aware of the layers of any one experience; when you notice your body, your breath, your feelings, your memories or imaginings.

Somatic movement education helps us focus on the detail, where the pattern of movement organises itself, in terms of weight, space, dynamics and relationships. However, somatic movement education is not only about understanding with our rational mind, it is also an attitude of permission, acceptance and non-judgement.

This book is an invitation to awaken your own somatic awareness, that of your body and your baby through play and exploration. Remain curious about what moves you, how you relate, express and organise this. You might find the following useful:

- Become more consciously aware of your own observation skills: how do you notice things? Where can you start to pay attention to the detail of the feeling of moving, without necessarily needing to interpret or know what movement 'means'?
- Try changing pace: slow some things down or speed some things up.
- Surprise yourself by moving in new ways: going beyond what is habitual or familiar can offer new experiences.
- Take your time and take care of the feelings that arise. Although all your feelings are welcome, we know that not all of them are easy to be with. Some require a conversation, while others just need some time for you to attend to yourself – so go have that bath, write, draw, be creative. If that is too big an ask, just be kind to yourself and seek out the support of others as best serves you.

Always remember that you are enough, you do not need to strive: how you are is welcome.

INTRODUCTION

Welcome to parenthood.

We all do it differently and this book celebrates that fact. Rather than tell you 'what' to do, I want to focus on the principles of baby development in a way that will help you understand your particular baby better, so that you can respond to their individual needs in your own way, with ease and confidence, right from the very start and have a joyful experience of parenthood.

The focus of this book is the first three months of your baby's life. It's a distinct period of time, often termed the 'fourth trimester', in which each of you is processing the birth experience you shared and acclimatising to a new way of being. It's a transitional phase, in which you might expect a few ups and downs, but for far too many parents the first few months feel more like a tornado has hit them. Emotions run high, low or so fast you just feel numb. It can be messy and uncomfortable one minute and a loved-up cuddle-fest the next. You lack sleep and lose perspective and the instincts you were relying on to tell you what to do can be difficult to access. Thinking straight is not really on the agenda, with tearful hormonal shifts surprising you in the first days and weeks. And while this is going on for you, your baby is also trying to cope with a new state of being. He is totally tuned into everything around him, and so connected to you that he does not yet realise where his body ends and yours begins. So if you are feeling out of balance, and out of your depth, he is right there in the thick of it with you. An unhappy baby will make their feelings very clear and soon no one is enjoying themselves at all. It doesn't have to be this way, and this book takes you one step further than most towards a more pleasant, confident and easy transition into parenthood.

We will look at a key question: What does my baby need in order to thrive, and how do they show me they need it? Because once you can understand what your baby is asking for, it becomes so much easier to provide it. Once you can perceive your baby's interests and priorities, you start to understand his developing personality and your bond with your baby evolves and deepens. The stronger your bond, the more attuned and responsive you are to his needs. This helps to establish the environment for your baby to form a secure attachment, which is one of the foundations of mental health and wellbeing.[1] Giving your child what they need, when they need it, is important. Unfortunately, as simple as it sounds, it may not always feel so easy when those needs are at odds with your own, and so the internal struggle of parenthood begins. This is where the approach that I describe can really make a difference to your life.

I have organised this book around general themes you will be dealing with as a parent: emotional regulation, touch, movement development, play and the routine activities of feeding and sleep, so that you can easily focus on specific topics you are curious about. Each theme includes exercises which aim to offer you resources as you deal with the demands of your role. The exercises bring your awareness to physical sensations in order to gain knowledge, insight and effect change, processes we work with in what is known as somatic movement education.[2]

The exercises will help you meet the practical demands of looking after a newborn. They are simple, short and manageable and the more you do them, the more effective they are. Just five minutes spent attending to your breath will bring you energy and refresh you when you are tired. Becoming aware of the support of gravity can help you calm down from being overwhelmed. Sensing and attending to your physical and emotional discomfort without judgement will help you look after yourself and therefore your child.

There are also movement explorations that will explain the principles your baby is learning for you to enjoy. These are integral to the process that I am guiding you through in the pages of this book: the skill of seeing the world from your baby's perspective as well as your own. You see, understanding babies is about understanding the primacy of movement in our developmental processes. And in this case, understanding means more than reading and thinking, which we are accustomed to as adults.

No amount of text can replace the felt experience of exploring a movement, sensing the responses that it elicits in your own body and mind and allowing this embodied perspective to inform your perception of your baby's activity. Finding comfort on the floor, gently moving through the movements your baby is mastering, will clarify what they are doing and what they may need to support them in their investigations. Mirroring your baby is a wonderful way of communicating your support and attentiveness directly to your baby. At a time when emotions and hormones are swinging like a pendulum, taking a moment to be aware of your bodily sensations can help you regulate your own emotions and, in so doing, you physically model the process of self-soothing. Our babies do not understand the meaning of our words, but they read our bodies like professionals and our bodies express exactly how we really feel.

Baby language is body language, and the movements they make are not simply indicating that their brain and body are growing in form and function. Movement is about expression and communication and it is the only way a young baby has to make their desires known. When you tune into your child's wavelength, you can find a different kind of logic, a fuller sense of being, connected to intuition. This will enhance your interactions with your child. That is the magic of working with somatic principles.

The 'fourth trimester' is your time to confront your own expectations about your role as a parent. As you encounter the assumptions of those around you about what you should or shouldn't be or do, you may find yourself wondering if 'martyr' is a more appropriate word to use than 'parent'. But here's the thing: responding to your child's needs effectively does not have to mean ignoring your own. You may not be able to sleep for eight hours straight at night for a few months, or even longer, but you can find ways to make the disturbance less difficult, or perhaps ensure you have support at other times to nap for longer stretches. The skill of finding some kind of balance between all the family's needs demands flexibility and awareness. It consists of small everyday decisions that add up to the whole atmosphere of your family life: balance is a process, ever-changing, growing and developing along with your baby. Once you accept the fluidity of the process you can relax and enjoy it.

So join me: read this book either when you are pregnant or once your baby has arrived (or read it twice!). Let it inspire and inform your thinking, let it relax and awaken your body awareness. When you have time, try out some of the games and activities I suggest. Notice how they make you feel, notice how your baby responds and build your own understanding of their temperament. When life is full of cuddles and kissing games, let me remind you of the value and importance of just hanging out with your baby, and when the skies are a bit more stormy use the information to calm the wind and rain and let the sun shine through again.

Let's begin with a question: What are your expectations of what it will be like to care for a baby? If you are one of the many people who have spent little or no time with a newborn baby, then you are really going into unknown territory. So I thought we would start by letting some new mums speak for themselves. I posted the question on a local Facebook group* and here are some of the responses I got...

I honestly thought my baby would sleep all day and I'd have time to go the museum, read a book, work out – ha ha. I've only managed to read two books since Oscar was born... sigh... and he's almost two! Juliana

Those first three months were the hardest, loneliest and most overwhelming experience of my life, even with the support of my wonderful husband. I thought the hard part would never end, but it did, and then it got amazing. Sarah

The only time I found it hard was when I listened to other people rather than my baby. Andrea

Time is relative and Zombies are real! Anna

Not all first time babies are challenging... You can get lucky! My baby slept for 16 hours per day, ate really well and was a dream in the first three months! Stephanie

It's not always love at first sight. And if it isn't don't feel bad that it takes you a moment longer to realise how much love you are actually capable to give and feel. Imke

Endless nights, and months that pass without you noticing. Agonising boredom, and hours spent enraptured just by her face. Crippling isolation, and the most profound connection I've ever experienced. Katie

---

* With thanks to the first-time mums from the ExpatBabies Berlin Facebook Group

I just felt useless. My (first) baby wouldn't stop crying.
I'd had this idea – this happy little fantasy – she'll know
I'm her mother, and that'll naturally comfort her, and
she'll hush. Nope. In the end, I just accepted all I could
do was be with her while she cried. Then one day, it
passed, and she started smiling. Thank fuck. Laura

What do these responses tell us? We are individuals, and so are our babies. There are so many factors that affect how your baby behaves in the first few months, and how you feel, that we can never predict your individual response. But whether your baby cries a lot or not at all, new parents tend to spend a lot of time worrying. Anxiety is a phenomenon that links us all: the sudden realisation of how total your responsibility is and how little experience you have in the practical care of a tiny baby can surprise even the most proficient among us. It can send you hunting through books and the internet day and night to work out what you should be doing.

Stop right there. Just for a moment, and focus instead on *yourself*. You see, the very first concern your baby has is that they are safe, and if you are panicking then 'safe' is definitely not the message they will be getting from you.

Remember that as an adult you are already skilled at regulating your emotions, and do it. Breathe deeply, listen to relaxing music, get a cuddle from a friend or loved one, talk to someone, take a bath. Then read on…

A note on the exercises

The explorations and somatic awareness exercises that I invite you to experience in this book are suitable for everyone, including pregnant and postnatal women with any level of movement experience or fitness, because you are always moving within your own comfort zone. If you have any concerns at all, check with your physician or health professional – show her or him the exercises so that they are aware of what they involve.

The somatic awareness exercises and relaxations become more effective the more often you do them, so if you can incorporate them into your daily routine, you will feel their effects grow. A perfect time to listen to them is when you feed your baby. To make it easier to practise you can download MP3s that will talk you through the explorations at **www.pinterandmartin.com/understanding-babies**.

1

LESS IS MORE:
EMOTIONAL REGULATION AND
DEVELOPMENT

Each little human organism is born a vibrating, pulsating symphony of different body rhythms and functions, which coordinate themselves through chemical and electrical messages... In the early months of life, the organism is establishing just what the normal range of arousal is, establishing the set point which its systems will attempt to maintain. When things drop below or rise above the normal range of arousal, the systems go into action to recover the set point or normal state. But first the norm has to be established, and this is a social process. A baby doesn't do this by himself but coordinates his systems with those of the people around him.[1]

Sue Gerhardt, *Why Love Matters*

Even a calm and gentle birth is an intense experience, a delicate negotiation between two minds and bodies requiring stamina, strength and a coordination of effort and release. However much the birth may feel like the completion of a process for you, for your baby it is just another challenge along the long road ahead. Only a year or so in the future that tiny newborn all snuggled in your arms will be a walking, babbling toddler – they have a long way to go and they are ready for it.

This little baby is neurologically primed to learn. She will learn from every experience she has, every position you hold her in, every mood surrounding her, every touch, sight, sound, smell and taste that she senses. The brain, as philosopher Alva Noë puts it, is the organ that will 'coordinate our dealings with the environment'.[2] The very activity of living – her interactions with the environment and people surrounding her – will cultivate your baby's brain development, creating the millions of neural connections that will later be pruned down until only the strongest and most individually useful remain. Your ability to respond effectively to her needs and mediate the drama inherent in her daily life is the key that will ensure this little brain, and indeed this little baby, will flourish. Science and common sense agree on this simple tenet: we thrive when we feel safe and contented, when we are loved and cared for sensitively. Before she can fully engage with the world, your baby has to feel safe and happy simply being in it.

If you read any books about child development you will sooner or later come across the term 'secure attachment' as something you should be striving to ensure for your child. The term was coined in the 1960s by psychologist John Bowlby, and the research was expanded in the 1970s by Mary Ainsworth as a way of categorising how children relate to their caregivers. The researchers devised the now famous 'strange situation' experiment, in which the child and mother are playing in a room. First a friendly stranger enters the playroom, and after a short time the mother leaves the room for a few minutes, so the child is alone with the stranger. The mother returns, the stranger leaves and after a while the mother exits the room, leaving the child completely alone for a few minutes. Researchers observed how the children related to their mothers when they left and returned and came up with different categories of attachment behaviour.

'Secure attachment' describes a child who will express their emotions when distressed and also express their excitement and pleasure on their mother's return. If they are distressed their mother will be able to help them calm down relatively easily. This is a child who feels safe with their parent and is able to express their feelings, trusting that they will be heard, soothed and helped by the adult. Adults who are able to regulate their own emotional state, who are responsive caregivers and attuned to their children's emotional needs, will be supporting their child to develop a secure attachment style.

Insecure attachment styles are either 'anxious-avoidant' or 'anxious-resistant'. In the anxious-avoidant category the child will seem very independent, and will ignore the mother's departure and return. However, when researchers tracked the children's heart rates, they showed that the departure of the mother was just as stressful for them as for the securely attached children: they had just learned not to express those emotions.

This kind of attachment can be formed when parents don't respond to their child's needs, reject or ignore their baby's cues, or are emotionally remote or uninterested in their baby. If a baby's main carer is depressed and emotionally distant from their child, perhaps seeing to their physical needs but unable to engage socially, this kind of attachment might result.

The anxious-resistant child displays an opposite 'insecure' reaction: they become extremely upset, even before the mother has left the room, and once she returns they are hard to comfort, clinging to their mothers and either showing signs of resentment or helpless passivity. Often the experiment had to be cut short as the child's distress was so extreme. This group of children showed very high levels of stress. A parent who is inconsistent in their behaviour, sometimes responding but sometimes ignoring needs, whose interactions are insensitive and intrusive, 'taking over' a play situation and then dropping it when they are bored, even though the baby is still playing, for example, may contribute to this kind of attachment style developing.

The fourth style of attachment, 'disorganised' or 'disoriented' attachment, was recognised later when researchers observed that some of the insecurely attached children had a lack of coping skills. Their behaviour on their mother's return was very inconsistent: sometimes they approached and were clingy, sometimes they ran away. These children are the most severely stressed and disturbed. The kind of parenting associated with this style of attachment is often the result of adult issues with drugs, alcohol or mental health.

The 'strange situation' experiment was devised for children aged 12–24 months and explored mothers' relationships with their children, assuming (as was mainly the case at the time) that they were the primary caregivers. It has been repeated with fathers and children in various age groups and adapted in various ways in the years since. Psychologists have explored how childhood attachment styles affect our social engagement and our personal relationships throughout our lives, as well as how they affect the physiology of our brains and our ability to engage with learning in a school environment. There is a general consensus that a secure attachment is the key to your child's health and wellbeing throughout life.

A whole industry has grown up around this information, and the internet is full of articles that can leave you worrying about the slightest miscommunication that you may have had with your child. Has that time you walked out on her when she was wailing because you were desperate for the toilet, or the time when she screamed and cried for an hour in the middle of the night ruined your relationship with your child forever? New parents' anxiety levels can be through the roof, so let's get one thing straight. Secure attachment is formed over *time*. As the parent of a newborn you are right at the start of it all: there is time to learn. The consistency of your response to your baby is key, and that doesn't mean you have to get it right every time or that you have to conform to particular practices if they don't feel right for you. For example, babywearing may be a wonderful option for you and your baby, or it may feel uncomfortable and distress you. You do not have to wear your baby in order to have a securely attached child. The same goes for other parenting behaviours, including routines and co-sleeping. Not all babies are the same, and nor are all parents. There is no 'one right way' to guarantee a securely attached child.

As valuable as attachment theory is in bringing our attention to the need for an attuned and responsive attitude towards our babies, it has also been subject to criticism over the years for its seeming implication that a woman's role should be at home caring for a child. Like any piece of research it is inevitably rooted in its cultural norms. Not only did the original researchers assume that women were the primary caregivers, but also that family life reflected a 'nuclear family' model, which is not the reality for many cultures around the world where babies are raised in multi-generational families and cared for more communally in the early years. You will make your own decisions about who is going to care for your baby, whether parents, other family members or childcare professionals: the most important thing is that the adults that care for your baby form loving, responsive relationships with them. It really is that simple.

When I work with families they are often surprised that the very basic activity of soothing their baby is so integral to their baby's development. The term psychologists use for this skill you are teaching your baby is 'emotional regulation': it's a strange term, as it sounds a bit restrictive, as though you are teaching someone to restrict their capacity to feel, but it is actually rather liberating. The more confident you are in your ability to find your way back to a calm, relaxed state of being, the more able you are to fully embody the emotions you are feeling. Our ability to express our feelings without losing control, to enjoy the nice ones fully or allow unpleasant ones to run their course and dissipate, is intrinsic to our psychological resilience. Emotional regulation is a skill intrinsic to our ability to function. Coaching your child to modulate emotions is a parenting constant, spanning infancy, the dramatic emotional landscape of toddlerhood and then surprising you with a new intensity as your child reaches adolescence. It is a long-haul parenting activity and it starts in the womb.

So what about now, at the very start of your newborn's life? Figuring out how she shows you what she needs, and how you can respond effectively, is the first job, and it happens without the support of language. It's a physical thing: you will be watching her expressions, her movements, listening to the kinds of sounds she makes to show she is hungry, hates her wet nappy, or indeed hates it more when you lay her down to change it. You will observe what she does when she wants a new perspective on the world, a person to 'talk' to or cuddle, and how she tells you that it is all too much for her to take on board. As you work these things out you will also be helping your baby pace her level of excitement so she does not become overwhelmed and lose herself in a wave of emotion each time she encounters something new. Much of your time will be spent searching for the soothing strategies that meet both her needs and your capacity to provide them – the everyday business of rocking, singing or sitting quietly with your baby in a darkened room. The more consistently effective you are in this task of soothing, the easier it will be for your baby to establish the 'set point of arousal', as Sue Gerhardt puts it, at which she can be awake, alert and attentive in a relaxed and open way, ready to move into sleep if she is tired, or to get excited or upset for a while without getting stuck in either extreme. Helping your baby to find that place and move into and out of it easily not only makes life easier for your baby, but also for you. I think it is a good place to start, don't you?

Meeting your baby

What do you know of babies? Have you ever met a newborn before, or is your own baby the first one you will hold in your arms? What is it you expect from them? If you spent your pregnancy imagining your baby in a certain way, then you may be surprised when they look or behave differently. However, it's important to build a connection with your baby while you are pregnant, so go ahead: talk, imagine and dream about your baby – just keep your mind open. Be aware that babies can be cute little rosebuds all cuddled up, but they can also shout, burp, fart, screw up their faces and grumble (even while they sleep). They may have birthmarks and blemishes, and be covered in fine hair or creamy vernix (the waxy substance that coats their body in the womb). Their heads may be pointy or foreheads squashed and wrinkled like a commander from the Klingon empire. Alien-looking or picture-postcard pretty, your baby is wonderful and completely their own person right from the start. Personalities are pretty much evident too if you look for them. Some babies are chilled out and relaxed, while others are more wakeful and alert. Their womb and birth stories will have had an impact on how they behave. It is easy to get caught up in comparing your baby to others, but pretty much pointless. Life would be so dull if we were all the same. Your body has done a wonderful job of seeing to your baby's needs inside you, and now it's time to be more conscious about it. Your baby has expectations of you too, but how will you know what they need when they can't speak to tell you?

For many new parents there will be a time during the first weeks when you start to panic... the sudden realisation of how total your responsibility is and how little experience you have in the practical care of a tiny baby can surprise even the most proficient among us. It can send you hunting through books and the internet day and night to work out what you should be doing. Please stop right there, take a breath and understand that you have everything you need to make this easy. In fact the hormones racing around your body, the hormones that are making it difficult to think straight, are working for you, not against you. These hormones make you slow down, make your brain fuzzy and make you more inclined to just sit and watch your baby and start to observe how they show you what they need.

You will observe with your whole body and emotions,

not just your eyes and your logical brain. Your body will respond without your conscious effort: breasts start to feel fuller as your baby gets hungrier, you will feel sleepy while your baby feeds and settles, you may be anxious when they are in the arms of another for too long, or surprisingly overwhelmed and exhausted when even the most welcome visitors leave. This change in you is not permanent, so don't worry and don't fight it. It is designed to help you recover after birth and bond with your baby and it too will pass. All you need to complete the picture you get from your baby is a bit of general information about what is possible for your baby at this particular time to help you read their responses more accurately. Then you can adjust your behaviour according to developmental principles as well as your instincts. The trick is having the trust in yourself, the confidence to feel yourself into their situation.

Interoception – inward focus

While life outside the womb brings many new things into your baby's environment, it is easy to forget that there are also many changes going on inside her body. Imagine feeling the sensation of breath filling your lungs. Do you even know that your ribs will stop moving out and come back to centre once more to push the air out? All those new sounds, direct, unmediated by your bubble of water, are they harsh to your ears? Or how about hunger? She has never felt that disturbing emptiness before, nor indeed the way milk squirts and flows, sweet and warm, to make it better. Your baby's world is full of interest and when her attention is drawn inward it is important to respect her need for those moments of inner focus.

Yet parents often disrupt these moments, trying to call their baby's attention back into interaction because they want to continue to play, or are worried that there is something wrong with their child because they seem to space out. Some parents even think that this behaviour means that their baby doesn't like them! Please don't worry. What your baby is doing has nothing to do with her feelings for you. This perfectly normal pattern of engagement followed by inner focus is how your baby helps herself to pace and integrate her learning. She may be distracted by a sensation inside her body, hypnotised by a contrast of light and dark (the most alluring combination to her maturing eyes), or perhaps she is integrating her experiences. It's like when you read something profound or meaningful... and then find yourself looking away, perhaps repeating the sentence or applying the idea to a situation you are familiar with. Your baby's brain may not be functioning on a verbal level yet, but it is working very hard and each experience, each subtle variation perceived by her maturing senses, is noted and learned from.

To get a better idea of what this inward focusing might be like, I would like you to try the 'Being inside' exploration below. It's easiest to do if you listen to it (download the MP3 from **www.pinterandmartin.com/understanding-babies**), but if needs must, simply read through and pause to tune in to your sensations as you go. As with all the explorations, make sure you are comfortable and feel free to move and adjust your position as you listen. If your mind wanders off, just gently guide it back once you realise it has happened. Our minds can take a while to learn to focus in this way, but the more often you try, the easier it will be.

Exercise: Being inside – adult exploration

Find a comfortable position sitting or lying down.

Let your eyelids close. Focus on the physical sensations you experience.

Bring your attention to those parts of your body that are in contact with the surface you are resting on. Notice where the weight falls through your body. Notice the places that release their weight less easily. Imagine them releasing, welcomed by the support of the earth, drawn down by gravity.

Bring your attention to your breath. Feel the sensation of the air coming in through your nostrils, notice the speed, the temperature – is it different when you breathe it out again?

Become aware of how your body moves as you breathe. Notice the way the front and back of your body expand on the in breath and contract again on the out breath.

Notice the way your ribs swing out to the side as you breathe in and glide back into the centre as you breathe out.

Notice how your spine lengthens when you breathe in – reaching back and away from your centre at either end – it's a tiny movement, but it's there.

And when you breathe out again, notice how the spine curls forward at both ends, like the letter C.

Feel that gentle wave, that stretch and curl, so small it's like the glimmer of an idea, before the action happens. Can you imagine it?

Now let your attention be drawn to any other inner sensations – the beat of your heart, an area of discomfort or numbness – whatever calls your awareness today.

Focus in and notice what happens when your attention arrives in that place. What happens to the sensation?

Take some time to explore.

When you are ready to finish, bring your attention out to your whole body. Imagine every single cell filling up and expanding with the air on the in breath and then letting go, releasing on the out breath.

Feel yourself getting bigger on the in and smaller again on the out.

Feel any remaining tension build on the in breath and flow out of you down and away on the out breath – through every single cell...

As the tension leaves your body, allow your fingers and toes to wriggle, your spine to stretch and let your eyelids lift from your eyes.

Take a moment to move, stretch or shake out.

Consider how you are feeling now. Are you calmer, more relaxed, refreshed?

How much did you notice? Did it surprise you how much or maybe how little you were able to sense going on inside? Did it take a lot of effort to stay focused? Are you feeling any different now than you did before you started? If you managed to focus deeply even for a short time, can you imagine how disruptive it might feel to be distracted out of that state?

Inner focus, or interoception, is a time of learning and the first step towards building emotional resilience. When I am aware of how I feel I can accurately communicate this need to my caregiver. If they respond appropriately it strengthens our relationship and my feeling of safety and trust in the world around me. It also has a role to play in our growing understanding of our agency in the world: by taking a short 'time out' we can pace our own level of excitement, and we can change how we feel. And finally, it helps us start to develop our sense of self – our understanding that we are separate entities from the world around us, that this body is our body and ours alone.[3] During the 'fourth trimester' – the three months after birth – your baby will spend hours noticing the sensations within her body as she moves. She will start to notice that these sensations are absent when she sees someone else moving, and gradually realise that the sensation is a result of her own body moving. By the time of her three-month birthday she will recognise her own limbs, hands and feet as she kicks and reaches out, moving them with more intention to grasp and explore the environment and her own body. If you continually distract your baby while they are in their interoceptive state it will become overwhelming and frustrating for them and harder for them to return to it. So recognising it, valuing and protecting it, is important for your baby's intellectual and emotional development.

Recognising and supporting inner focus

Your baby may have a specific 'look' when they are focusing inwards, which you will get to know, but to start with look for moments when:

- Your baby's eyes are a bit unfocused. Perhaps they tend to drift to one side, or she looks a bit 'spaced out', as if she is awake but not really 'there'.
- She looks away or simply does not meet your gaze, just stares into space. Her torso is relaxed, her arms and legs may be moving gently, but she is not flapping in an excited or effortful way.

These moments of inner focus happen throughout your baby's awake time, when she senses a physical change within herself, for example the feeling of a full bladder or a change to her environment, like being moved to the changing table, or as part of any kind of playful exchange between you. When you notice your baby going into this mode give her some physical and emotional space. Let go of the game or pause the activity, avert your focus too, move your face further away and watch from a distance until she looks for you again. Depending on how sensitive family and friends are when they visit, you may find yourself having to intervene to protect your baby from overwhelm. I suggest pointing out what you see your baby doing and explaining that this is her way of showing that she needs a bit of space to understand or get used to what is happening. You are the person that knows your baby best, so you can help visitors to get to know her too.

The drama of the outside world

Inner experiences aside, there is also a whole lot going on outside and around your baby that will draw her attention and interest, and make her excited or scared. Apart from the natural drama inherent in all the 'first time' experiences on offer, the way your baby perceives the world around her makes her susceptible to emotional extremes. To cope with all this drama she has a brain that is about a third of its adult size. It is a work in progress and so are the nerves that bring information into it and carry the responses out into an action. This means that your baby needs extra time to register and experience and then to express her response. Dr Annie Brook, a perinatal psychologist and somatic therapist, suggests that a newborn will process information six to ten times more slowly than an adult.[4] I'm sure you will find yourself naturally slowing down when you deal with your baby, because you have recognised this fact without even thinking about it. It is especially important to pay attention to when you want to change something about your baby's environment or position.

Imagine you have just fed your baby on the sofa and you need to change her nappy.

- Get your baby's attention – make eye contact or place the palm of your hand on her belly. PAUSE and wait until she is really attending to you.
- Speak to her, tell her what is happening. PAUSE and notice if your own body is ready to move.
- Stand up, PAUSE and feel your own balance, and then slowly walk over to where you will change her. PAUSE and take a moment to check you have everything you need to hand.
- Put her down, while maintaining as much body contact as possible. Bend over with your baby and slowly lower her to the mat, head going down last. PAUSE and notice how your baby is responding. When she starts to settle, slowly slide your hand out from under her head, perhaps placing it on her belly again to reassure her if she starts to show distress, until she is calm before proceeding.

And so on…

With each pause you will notice your baby's attention going inward and then out again in anticipation. Each time your baby is attending they are learning: how is this surface different from the last one? Can I push away more easily or do I sink? What sounds or smells are here? Oh, that shadow looks interesting. That pattern is familiar… and so on. You are teaching, they are learning and you thought you were simply changing a nappy!

Of course, as the weeks go by and routines become familiar you will speed up, and your baby's response times will get faster too. But this principle is very useful to remember if you are tempted to rush through something because your baby is upset and you think that the quicker it is over the better. It may be the speed that is part of the issue. Sometimes by slowing yourself down you will be able to prevent overwhelm from escalating. It can also help you recognise a detail in your actions that is contributing to your baby's upset, for example that you are moving your baby's head later than their body and this is startling them when you lift them and making them cry.

How your baby takes the world in

Now let's take a look at how your newborn senses the world outside, because it is a bit different from the way our adult sensory perception works. Your baby is born with the sense of *touch* in first place in terms of maturity: it is of such primary importance that it gets a chapter all of its own (Chapter 2) so let's move on to the others.

Hearing is also mature: your baby has been able to hear the sounds within you and outside your body for some months already. She is familiar with the voices and music she has listened to during your pregnancy. High-pitched, sing-song voices are most attractive to your baby and most adults tend to find themselves speaking to their little ones with at least some adaptation to their baby's preferences. The womb is not the quietest place to be, and while she may startle at a loud noise at first, she will learn to tune it out and ignore it over time.

Next on the list is *smell*: there have been experiments that show that a baby, even at only a few days old, prefers the smell of her mother, and in particular her mother's breastmilk, over another woman and another woman's milk. Tastebuds form early in foetal development and are tuned in to sweet tastes, preferring breastmilk to formula.

The least fully developed sense at birth is *vision*: the eyes need an environment more conducive to their function to help them learn to focus and track, discern proximity and all those other amazing things they do. At birth, your baby will see most clearly at a distance of around 20–25cm. However, rather like a short-sighted person without their glasses on, things that are further away will be a bit blurry. Your baby's gaze will be drawn to sharp contrasts: dark hair as it meets the hairline of pale skin, dark lips outlining teeth, or the black and white images that you will find on so many newborn toys. She cannot yet see all the colours, and controlling her gaze and tracking objects is a difficult task that she starts to manage during the first three months. If your baby's head and neck are supported horizontally, however, she will be able to turn her head to look at something that interests her right from birth. Lynne Murray and Liz Andrews, in their book *The Social Baby*,[5] have a lovely picture story of a baby just a few minutes old, gazing up at his mum and then turning his gaze towards his father when he hears him speak. Newborn babies prefer to look at faces and representations of faces right from the start. By the time your baby reaches eight weeks, colour vision is kicking in as well as an overriding desire for and interest in social interaction.

There is a magical period of social and emotional intimacy that arises around the end of the second month for an intense window of eight weeks or so. Identified as a period of 'core relatedness',[6] you will know it's happening when you realise you have just spent the last hour with your baby gazing at each other's faces. Your face and every micro expression that appears on it will be the most fascinating thing in your baby's world, and you will respond by mimicking her expressions, and having smile, grimace and tongue-poking 'conversations'. At around three months of age your baby may start to become interested in tracking toys and objects with her eyes and eventually reaching to try and grab them, and her world will be less blurry. By around five months her colour vision will be on par with an adult's, and by six months 20/20 vision will have arrived, although the eye and other aspects of vision continue to develop until around eight years of age.

While not all senses are fully developed at birth, it seems they know how to work together in a global way that is perfectly designed to provide babies' brains with the maximum amount of information about an object or experience. Research using brain imaging has shown us that 'the brains of babies and synesthetes share common features, it's possible that an infant's perception may look a lot like an extreme case of synesthesia.'[7] Synesthesia is defined as 'The production of a sense impression relating to one sense or part of the body by stimulation of another sense or part of the body', so the capacity to 'smell' a colour, or 'hear' a physical touch. If our babies experience the world in this multi-sensory way, if the kiss on their forehead brings music to their ears, or the hum of your lullaby floods their inner eyes with colour, no wonder over-stimulation is so easy.

This cross-utilisation of the senses does not end with the way babies *experience* the world. It also plays a part in how they *explore* it. Your baby can translate abstract experiences from one sensory modality to another. One experiment that demonstrates this facility involved providing blindfolded babies with a pacifier that had a particular shaped teat to suck. When the baby was later shown this pacifier alongside another, differently shaped one, they looked at the pacifier they had experienced more intently and more often than the other one, indicating recognition.[8] So the baby could translate their *felt* experience into *visual* perception. And it's not just a particular link between vision and touch: this 'amodal perception' relates to all the senses. It is hardly surprising that your baby's world is a dramatic one. Your baby is drawn to the drama – the intensity of a moment, a contrast of colour, a change of pace, motion, pitch or volume. She is totally attentive, at one with the world and completely open to everything around her. From the emotional tone of the conversations that she hears, to the tension or comfort level of the arms that hold her. It is hardly surprising then that overwhelm is the issue you will spend most of your time dealing with in these first few months. So setting that baseline state of arousal we talked about earlier can take some work on your part.

Let's look now at the practical tools that may help you in your task.

Reading the signs of overwhelm

Your baby will get upset. It's part of life. Recognising why your little one is crying and helping them is often the hardest part of parenting a newborn, because it upsets you so much too.

When your baby cries, you need to work out why. Recognising hunger is pretty straightforward. Apart from the fact that you know when you last fed your baby, if you stimulate the mouthing reflex by stroking the side of your baby's mouth gently and she turns towards your touch and opens her mouth, she is definitely ready for a feed. Environmental issues like bright lights, sudden noises or strong smells, feeling too warm or cold or needing a fresh nappy can all be identified and responded to. A simple cry to get your attention and bring you to her should be easily silenced by your presence and your patience as she takes a bit of time to realise you are there and respond.

Crying for no practical reason can often be a sign of overwhelm. It's a good idea to start to identify how your baby shows you that she is starting to feel over-stimulated before it even gets to the crying stage. There are several things to look out for:

- Your baby may close her eyes or turn her head or gaze away.
- Hiccups.
- Your baby may start to wriggle or squirm, frown, or look uncomfortable.
- Your baby may flap her arms and legs in an excited way, with eyes wide open: it seems like she is having fun at first glance, but she can easily tip from excitement to distress.
- Your baby may simply start to shout or cry all of a sudden.

Take time to notice what your baby's signals are: she will have a preference. Respond by giving her space or taking her away from the stimulating situation. This can be tricky, and often we don't notice what is wrong because we are part of that situation and caught up in the emotion of it ourselves. Sometimes, if the situation involves others, it can feel socially difficult to remove ourselves and our baby from the source of stimulation.

In my classes we practise simply observing our babies: either holding them, or watching them as they lie next to us, and noticing the small movements they make: their expressions, their speed or slowness, the quality of their movement – is it flowing or jerky, effortful or effortless? It can be helpful to take a few minutes every day to simply witness your child without interacting, just observing. When you learn to notice the details in a restful mood, then you will find it easier to see what changes in a situation when overwhelm begins.

We also practise describing what we see – without making value judgements – and this is a skill that can help you out of those tricky moments when your relatives are ramping up the excitement and you want to prevent it turning to tears. Simply pointing out what you see and letting them know that this is how your child shows it is all getting a bit too much for her can help. For example, you could say 'Oh look Mum, see how Mia has started blinking and her little hand is moving up and down? That usually means she is getting a little over-excited, and she is just about to get upset – perhaps we can…' Notice that there is no blame, just information, so no one can really be offended by your intervention.

When babies cry

We are not meant to find it easy to 'let' our babies cry. Indeed, although tears are one way of ridding the body of the stress hormone cortisol, it seems that crying and distress raise the level of cortisol in the brain to levels which, if high and present for long periods of time, can cause physical damage. Avoiding overwhelm and attending to practical needs promptly can help keep reasons for your baby to cry to a minimum, and yet cry they will. How else can this little person tell you that she is feeling sad, or bored, or perhaps a bit anxious? Crying is one of the only ways your baby can express her emotions. She isn't able to complain with words or even make a wide range of expressive grumble sounds, so from time to time she will undoubtedly cry.

For many parents this is so distressing that they swoop in and instantly hush, rock, distract or feed their babies in order to stop the tears as fast as possible. And that is totally understandable. However, when you do this every single time your baby cries, there are two messages that you are communicating. Firstly, your reaction suggests that this is an emergency situation and you, the parent, are distraught about it too. The implication is that no one can cope with this. Secondly, that your baby needs to be quiet. Expressing negative/sad emotions is not appropriate.

Let's transpose this to an adult situation. A friend comes over, obviously upset about something that has just happened. She starts to explain what it is, but before she finishes her first sentence you rush up and give her a big hug, and start making shushing sounds. Then, as she raises her voice so that you can hear what happened, you grab an apple from the fruit bowl and start trying to push it into her mouth! How does your friend feel? How would you feel?

But it's different with babies, isn't it, that feeling that you are the only one that can help? So how do we help most effectively? The answer is by responding in a calm way, by taking a few moments to work out what is wrong, and if there is nothing that you can practically do, like feed or move her, hold her and simply *listen* for a moment. Make sure your baby is aware of your presence and empathy. Listen before you respond, breathe deeply yourself, stay calm and watch for a minute: you may well see her start to settle down again.

If your baby is not already calming down in response to your presence, your voice and your attention, then try to soothe her with whatever method feels appropriate for you. Stay with that for some time to give your baby time to show its effect on her… remember that her nervous system is still a work in progress. If that is still not the answer you can try another strategy, but always give it plenty of time and if you can bear to simply stop and be with her for a few minutes before you transition to the next rocking or singing attempt to soothe, all the better. If she is starting to feel overwhelmed by all these changes this will give her a chance to compose herself. Just the simple act of sitting quietly with her in a darkened room may be all she needs to relax again.

As your baby matures, letting her know that big emotions are okay and that expressing them is how you let them run their course is an important lesson she will learn through experience. It takes confidence on your part and the ability to hold that emotional space for your baby. Your empathic yet calm presence is vital when she is upset. It signals that it is not the end of the world, that her emotions will pass and everything will be alright again. It can be really hard work for parents to just stay present and aware, ready to help when action is needed rather than frantically doing anything possible to make that crying sound stop. I know what it's like, and I've been there myself, but you will be giving your baby a chance, just for a moment or two, to express her feelings and then she may find that they are gone and she starts to feel better again all by herself. I have watched as a four-month-old, held in his mother's arms, with her full attention on him, had a little cry, paused, listened to her commiserate, cried a minute more and then took a deep breath, closed his eyes and fell to sleep with a smile on his face. You will learn when you need to give your baby space and when you need to act fast to bring calm as you get to know your baby better.

The fundamentals of soothing

At the heart of whatever way you choose to soothe your newborn is your attitude. The more relaxed and able to 'contain' the enormous overwhelming emotion that your baby is experiencing you are, the faster your baby will be able to process it and calm down again. If you are panicking, if your face is screwed up in anxiety as you try to work out what is wrong, if your body is tense or you are crying along with her, your own overwhelm will distress your baby even more. Try one of the ideas in 'Peace in the storm' below to help you, or ask a calmer person to take your baby while you collect yourself.

Exercise: Peace in the storm – ways to help yourself stay calm while soothing your child

When you hear your baby stir, place your hand gently on her belly. Now focus on your own breath. Breathe in and feel your face, neck and shoulders fill up and expand, then breathe out and feel the breath flowing down though your body and into the floor, taking any tension with it. Let the sound of her crying wash over you like a wave in the distance.

If you are holding or rocking your little one and they are crying, focus on your breath and your connection to the floor. Let the sound of their cry fade from the foreground of your mind and focus in on your own body. Release your shoulders, your face. Deepen and slow your breath. Check in with your baby, tell them that they will feel better again soon. If you know what has upset them then explain it to them and tell them (if you truthfully can) that it is not so bad, and they will get used to it. Tell them you are here and with them and all will be well again. Be sensitive to the rhythm of their cry, pausing so they have a chance to express themselves too.

Explaining to your baby what you are doing to calm them can help you stay focused and calm. Like a mantra, for example. 'I'm rocking you gently, side to side, mmm mmm, side to side to sleep.' Of course your baby doesn't understand the meaning of your words, but intention comes through in your tone and your inflection and will help you really feel that calmness and reassurance for yourself.

Remember, you are still that metaphorical womb: you offer the boundary, the assurance that the distress will not get out of control, because you won't let it. Whatever soothing method feels right to you is the one to go for. Over the coming weeks you will start to see your baby's preferred ways of soothing and you will come up with some creative and entirely personal ways of handling them. The important thing is to take it slowly.

The first principle to think of is familiarity: she has spent most of her life inside you, so anything that may remind your baby of the sensation of being in the womb should help her feel safe again. Here are the basics, but adapt and use the principles to create your own specific approaches – that's part of the fun of parenthood.

Soothing strategies

Connect then respond

Most babies don't suddenly start wailing – there is some kind of build-up, be it squirming physically or a loud cry or two. The quicker you can get to your child and acknowledge their need the better. What can make a difference is your behaviour at that point: if you can stay relaxed, let your baby know you are there and be ready to find out what is wrong; if you place your hand on her, speak to her softly and let her respond to your voice, you will be offering her a way out. She may be able to tune into your calmness rather than allow the emotion to overtake her. Remember your baby has no other way to tell you 'I'm getting a bit hot in this blanket' or to ask if there is anyone around because she's a bit bored. Not every cry is a calamity, but it will become one if you add to the emotion of the moment.

Curl up to calm down

If your baby is crying or unsettled try reminding them of the support of the womb by curling her up into a ball shape when you hold her. Cuddle your baby close with her knees bent and her back in the 'C' position, head supported so it doesn't fall back and elicit the startle reflex. Keep your cuddle flexible, so if your child stretches out let her feel the resistance of your arms and body, but allow her body to move yours. Stay in contact physically while offering more space. Then, when you feel her body start to relax again, support her to curl up even more.

Dancing in the dark

Remember at the end of your pregnancy how, when you were finally in bed or resting, your baby would decide to dance around and keep you awake? Well the inverse of that, when you were busy in the day and moving around and she was still, gives you a clue about why all that rocking and swinging and jiggling can help. It's what she is used to, it's familiar. Keep your baby's head supported and moving with her spine for safety. A useful position to try is holding her, tummy against your chest, head on your shoulder and your arm along her back, cupping her head. Move gently and steadily (avoid shaking), keeping the rhythm for about three minutes. If it doesn't seem to be working, try a different motion, rhythm or another soothing strategy.

Sitting on one of those big gym balls while you do this may be helpful if you are tired and standing up feels hard. The closer you hold your baby to the centre of your torso, the lighter she will feel. All kinds of movements can work: quite surprising big ones as well as gentle, slow and steady. And remember, stick to one movement for a few minutes before you change... less is more.

Soundscapes

Your baby is used to the sounds she heard in the womb. The whooshes, the heartbeat, your voice, songs that you may have heard or sung. Stand next to the washing machine or dishwasher as they do their thing, play some music, sing to her, hum or swoosh... all these can help, but again, pick one and stick with it for a while before you change or stop. Let me sound a note of caution about your musical choices. Some babies can be very sensitive to music: my second child, for example, cried every time we played music in a minor key. However calm and relaxing I found the music, he would simply start to wail. It took us a few days to realise what the problem was, but once we did and changed our playlists he was happy and so were we.

Modelling behaviour

Mirror neurons are a wonderful thing, and rather like the idea of relaxing your body so your baby feels more relaxed, you can use your breathing and your voice to help your child calm down. My husband was a master of this technique. He would simply hold our babies with their belly on his chest (in an upright position), sway softly and then start breathing regularly and deeply. Sometimes he would even softly mimic the sounds they were making in time to his breath and then start to slow them down and bring them into a lower register until he was simply gently humming. Often they would simply tune into what he was doing and follow his lead until they were calm or even asleep.

Baby hammock, blanket or fabric rocker

If you are stressed out, tense or upset and unable to pass your baby to someone else to help her to calm down, equipment like a baby hammock can be very useful. You can also simply place her on a blanket or large scarf, pick up the corners and rock her in it: as you pick her up she will tend to roll into a fetal position naturally. Make sure you raise her head off the ground before the rest of her body, and lower it last to avoid the startle reflex. I regularly use 2.5m lengths of coloured organza in my classes for this with babies of four weeks and older. They are often mesmerised by the fact that the whole world has changed colour and yet they can still see their parent or caregiver due to the transparency of the fabric. A long piece of fabric means you can relax your arms and shoulders as you rock them (they don't need to be far from the floor to benefit from the swaying motion) and the way the fabric moulds to their body reminds them of the safety of the uterine walls.

Suckling

Suckling at the breast or using a pacifier have been strategies for soothing since babies began. The act of suckling releases the love hormone, oxytocin, which makes us feel calm and relaxed. Suckling activates our parasympathetic nervous system, lowers the heart rate, sends blood to the internal organs to help them digest and limits adrenaline and cortisol levels in our system.[9] In short, it works.

However, it is not always possible, easy or even desirable to provide your child with something to suckle. Nipples can get tender and sore after hours of comfort-suckling, and a mum with a baby constantly attached to the breast can feel trapped, resentful and incredibly tired. This is why most baby care advice emphasises the need to discourage your baby from sleeping with a nipple in her mouth. It may not be as easy as it sounds, as newborns will often fall asleep while feeding. Pre-empting that by gently popping your finger in their mouth to break the vacuum they create as they drop off may mean your baby wakes, and soothing them back to sleep in another way may well be necessary.

While part of falling asleep at the breast is about the warmth, love and full belly you provide, using a pacifier can also satisfy your baby as the oxytocin response is the same. They bring pros and cons with them, as you might expect. Unless otherwise advised by a medical practitioner, you should wait to introduce a pacifier until breastfeeding is well established and your baby is gaining weight steadily. People often feel very strongly about pacifiers, but if you have a baby who is insistent on suckling they can be life-saving, so inform yourself and keep your mind open to the possibility of their use.[10]

Some babies come into this world as hand and finger-sucking pros, as it can be a favourite pastime in the womb, which is great except for the fact that they may not be able to find their hands easily for a few weeks. Swaddling your baby with their elbows bent so that their hands are near their faces can help them achieve their desire.

Forming soothing habits

Someone will say it: 'You don't want them to form a habit!' or the more traditional, 'You're making a rod for your own back if you let her do that!' They are probably right to an extent, in that we all have habits. I bet there are certain things you tend to do when you feel stressed. Perhaps you go for a run, take a hot bath, grab a drink or something to eat or ring your best friend. The same goes for your baby, so when you find a soothing strategy that works you are very likely to have to stick to it for some time. Make sure you offer your baby support that you can physically sustain. Nipple suckling is an example: it may be easier to just let your baby sleep while suckling now, but after three months you might be tearing your hair out. Similarly, rocking your baby to sleep may be fine when they weigh 3kg, but when that has tripled it's not so much fun. If mixing it up and offering different soothing methods at different times seems to frustrate your child, you might need to get creative and adapt your method to suit you better, for example putting a mattress in the kitchen or utility room so you and your baby can at least lie down while the washing machine whirrs and whooshes beside you and lulls her to sleep. If it's possible for you, you could consider investing a bit of cash to make your soothing strategies easier. The rocking chair I bought when expecting my third child saved my 42-year-old tired body: it was one of those glider chairs, with a foot stool, and I could rest while he slept on my chest. It was a lifesaver in those first few months. Remember that however silly these adjustments may seem, what matters is that they make your life easier. Don't worry, you won't be stuck with a mattress in the kitchen forever: babies' development goes in phases, and their preferences change – this too will pass.

One last word before we move on. If you're yet to have your baby and are perhaps feeling a bit freaked out by this barrage of detailed information about something so obvious as calming your baby, or your baby is already here and you have been exploring the subtleties of soothing for some time – just keep in mind that whatever way you soothe your baby needs to work to soothe you too. If you are standing there rocking her while your brain works overtime, desperate for her to sleep so you can go get on with something, you are missing a trick. The 24-hour job of parenting a newborn is so much easier if you look after yourself and allow that rocking, that mantra, that slow comfortable suck to lull you into a restful place too. It may not enable you to sleep, but at least you can close your eyes and clear your mind, breathe deep and remember that everybody, even that babe in your arms, has to sleep eventually. You may not get exactly what you want, but you will have a little bit more energy.

2

A TOUCH OF LOVE

Depending upon how you look at it, the skin is the outer surface of the brain, or the brain is the deepest layer of the skin. [1]

Deane Juhan, *Job's Body*

Have you ever wondered why it is that a squeeze of the hand can reassure you, or the hug of a good friend can make you suddenly feel so safe and warm inside? Have you ever jumped or flinched with surprise when someone brushes past you unexpectedly? Touch is so fundamentally important to us that the tactile or somatosensory system is the first to form and the most fully developed of all our senses at birth.

In the adult world we tend to think of touch as additional to our words. It's different for your baby: there are no words they understand for a touch to augment. So for your baby the nature of the touch itself, the caress of your hand, the welcome of your body, the textures and surfaces they encounter are intensely noticed. A newborn's brain is not ready to understand the things you say, but it is fully primed to read the subtleties of tension, tone and emotion that your body communicates unconsciously though physical contact. What you communicate through the quality of your touch is more important than the cooing sounds or calming words you may be saying as you do it: those are more helpful as a way of keeping yourself relaxed.

Touch experience has an effect: not only on our baby's emotions, but also on their physical body, their growth rate, their health, digestion and their developing intellect. Holding your baby close, caressing them – in fact, every loving, physical interaction you have – is vital to their development. In the film *The Moving Child*,[2] Dr Bruce Perry, psychiatrist and child trauma specialist, says 'we know that in infants touch and the opportunity for motor activity are as important for the physical growth of the brain as calories.' That's right: touch, as well as movement, is fundamental to the volume and structure of the brain, as fundamental as the milk your baby drinks! That is nothing short of amazing. So it's lucky that our instinct is to cuddle and hold, carry and caress our newborns. While it may be pleasurable for you, you are never 'just' holding the baby, you are supporting their physical health and emotional resilience for the rest of their lives by attending to one of their most fundamental developmental needs.

In this chapter we are going to look at it all; how far the scientists have come in explaining the effect of touch and what somatic practice can add to our understanding. I will discuss the kinds of touch experience your newborn baby will expect from you and offer practical tips to ensure you and your baby comfortably enjoy their benefits. You will discover what you can learn if you 'listen' with your hands and how to offer support through this gentle physical awareness. Massage is on our list too, with easy ways to introduce this ancient art to your baby from the very first. And I'll address what happens if your baby does not seem to welcome your touch as you expect, or you are finding it hard to offer loving touch, and feeling disconnected or irritated by long hours of holding your little one. I will help you consider the reasons why this may be the case, and offer simple, effective strategies to address it, as well as discussing where you can go for specialist support if you need it.

So sit back comfortably and notice the sensations you feel on your skin right now: the brush of fabric, the weight of your body sinking into its support, the temperature of the air around you. Feel how the world is touching you at this moment in time. Now take one deep breath in... and slowly out. Let's begin.

Science and touch

So why is it that the sensations we feel at the very periphery of our bodies have such a major structural and functional importance to our whole being? Let's go back to the quotation at the beginning of the chapter, which characterises the skin, our largest organ, as part of the brain itself. This connection is established early in our development when we are comprised of just three 'germ' layers of cells: the ectoderm and endoderm, present from around 12 days after conception, joined a little later by the mesoderm, which forms in between the two. These three germ layers create all the tissues and structures with in our bodies. It is the ectoderm that gives rise to our central nervous system (spinal cord and brain) and our outermost layer, the skin. Skin and brain are essentially made of the same stuff.

As the tissues and structures differentiate and develop, the part of the ectoderm that will become the skin moves outwards to accommodate the growth of tissue and structures within the body. The cells that will become the spinal cord and brain become enclosed within the developing vertebrae and skull bones, maintaining their central position within the body. Despite this increasing physical distance, the connection between skin and brain is set to continue along the nerves. Nerves are essentially bundles of elongated cells we call neurons which run parallel to each other from any area of the body into the spinal cord and into the brain. There are various types but essentially they do one of two things: sensory nerves tell our spinal cord and brain what is happening within and outside our body, and motor nerves tell us how to respond to whatever is going on. Each of these nerve cells is coated along its length by myelin, a fatty substance that both protects the nerve and enables messages to move quickly along the fibre so that our responses are appropriate and timely.

We are born with brains about one-third of their adult size, equipped with almost our total quota of neurons already formed, and there are billions of them. However, not all of them are connected up to the brain yet, and many are not yet myelinated, making them slow to relay information back and forth. This is perceptible to us: we can see that babies are slower to express their responses than adults, as I discussed in the previous chapter. Over the next 18–24 months our neural plasticity is at its peak, as nerves make connections, link to particular areas of the brain, and the myelin sheaths spread out to surround them and increase their efficiency. We also begin to refine the architecture of the brain: those neurons that are least often used are pruned away until we are left with a bespoke nervous system suited to the life we lead.

So why is this important? Here we get to the 'touch promotion' bit. The connecting-up process actually begins at the skin end of the nerve, not, as was once assumed, at the brain end. So the frequency and nature of the touch we receive directly influences the structure and function of our nervous system and our brain. I'm sure we have all seen images of the foetus in utero, sucking their hands: it makes total sense that we should stimulate the mouth and lips well in advance so that our nerves are ready to coordinate the complex activity of feeding at birth. Consider also that every time we feed there is more stimulation. It is hardly surprising then that our babies choose to explore objects with mouth and lips rather than their fingers or their eyes for many months, as they get much more information that way! Thus touch helps us get information and respond more efficiently, by ensuring that our nerves develop strong, resilient connectivity. Touch is a major part of the processes that form our brain.

I started the chapter by reminding you of the emotional power of touch, so let's unpick for a moment why touch affects our emotions and how emotions cause physical changes in our body. Our sensory nerves send signals to two centres of the brain. First is the somatosensory cortex, which is all about facts: where have we been touched, in what fashion, how intense was the pressure and so on. Second is the posterior insula, which registers the emotional tone of the touch. As David Linden, professor of neuroscience at Johns Hopkins University School of Medicine, stated in a recent TED talk,[3] *there is no sensation without emotion*.

And that means everything: from the action of your stomach digesting its food, to the brush of your mother's lips on your forehead. Sensations that originate within our bodies and outside of them all have an emotional tone. When the touch we receive is loving, respectful and welcome, our brain produces endorphins. These are opioid chemicals (that's right, love is addictive) and they make us feel happy, safe and secure. Our bodies work well in this state: blood circulates to our organs, and our minds are relaxed and able to take in new information with ease. We enter a parasympathetic state. However, as a response to unpleasant touch or when we are not held or touched enough, the opposite happens: we feel stressed, our brain responds by releasing cortisol and elevated levels of cortisol that persist for long periods of time affect physical growth, digestive and immune system function, intellectual ability and emotional development.

While all of this may feel like old news to you, it was as recently as the 1980s that scientists believed that babies did not feel pain, so operations and painful procedures were performed without any anaesthetic.[4] You may still find some professionals who tell you that babies don't feel pain as keenly as adults, even though the latest research[5] shows that they do feel it and that their pain threshold is lower than an adult's so they feel it sooner. Even kangaroo care, which is a protocol for the care of premature babies that recommends regular loving touch, skin-to-skin contact with parents or carers and gentle mobilising of limbs has not yet reached all hospitals as standard, despite many studies proving the beneficial outcomes.[6] Research knowledge is slow to feed through to actual practice, so it is important that you are aware of what is known, so that you can make well-informed decisions about your baby's care.

Let's take a short break from the theory here and do a little experiment that brings your awareness to the way your whole body communicates through the simple act of being in contact. You need to work with another person – this could be your partner, a friend or even an older child (it can be a nice way to start a conversation about what it might be like to live with a new baby). This exercise is easiest to do sitting on the floor. Make sure you are nice and comfortable, and if you can, download the audio track from **www.pinterandmartin.com/understanding-babies** to make it easier to follow.

Exercise: Exploring body language

1. Sit back-to-back with your backs touching lightly over as much of their surface as possible. It doesn't matter if legs are crossed or out in front of you, they should be relaxed and comfy.

2. Close your eyes and bring your attention to your own body. Feel the floor underneath you, feel the breath filling and emptying, feel your ribs floating out to the sides as you breathe in, returning to centre on the out breath. Notice any physical sensations or tensions within your own body – just notice.

3. Now allow your attention to move to the sensations you are feeling through your back. Notice the warmth or coolness, notice the movements of your partner's back as they breathe, notice the contact – where it falls, how it feels. What else do you perceive?

4. When you feel ready you can allow your contact to deepen, and take a moment just focused on your physical connection, leaning into each other so that your weight is evenly shared between you. A gentle rock forwards and backwards together will help you find a comfortable mid-point of balance.

5. Rest for a moment and then, both at the same time, very, very slowly and softly move away from the connection, staying aware of your

physical sensations as you go. Note how it feels to leave.

6. Take a couple of breaths and then share a few words about your experience.

When I take parents through this exercise, they are often surprised at just how much they can sense about their partner: the rhythm of breathing, the level of tension in their shoulders, areas of warmth and coolness and sometimes even their heartbeat. Some people find their breath slowing down or speeding up to synchronise with their partner's. Some people become quite emotional when they move apart again.

When you consider that your newborn is intensely focused on sensation, it is easy to see that the signals your body gives out when you hold him close will have a profound effect on his mood and the general levels of stress he encounters. Imagine how your baby will feel if your body is tense when you hold him, if you are sitting uncomfortably worried about moving your arm because you don't want to wake him, if you're hungry or you need the loo.

It is surprisingly easy to get stuck in discomfort with a young baby, focussed as you are on your baby's needs. They cry, you pick them up, you notice they have pooed, so you change their nappy and by this time their cries are quite intense so you just plonk yourself down in the nearest chair to feed them. You realise you need a drink but there is nothing within reach... the baby falls asleep, you try to move but they wriggle with displeasure so you just stay there suffering… or even if you manage to doze, you end up with a crick in your neck, aching shoulders or a desperate rush to the toilet when you come to again. Remember this: *comfort is key*. The more comfortable you are, the more comfortable and relaxed your baby will be. If you feel tense or uncomfortable your baby will feel it too. They may not respond the first time, but if it carries on throughout the day, you will have a stressed-out babe to deal with by the early evening. No fun for anyone.

Case study

A client came to see me with her eight-week old baby. She told me her daughter was unsettled all the time, frustrated and unhappy when lying on her tummy, bad at napping and generally a bit tense, especially when feeding.

As the session progressed the baby was hungry and the mother started to feed her. I noticed that she was sitting really uncomfortably, with no support under her elbows or behind her back. I invited her to sit against the wall and propped her up with cushions so her arms were supported and her head could rest back. I encouraged her to relax and breathe deeply.

As the mother relaxed, so did the baby. She started to suckle with a more regular rhythm, and mum said the suckling got stronger. When the baby was finished, she looked happy and satisfied, burped the moment mum held her up on her shoulder and lay contentedly in her mother's arms. She was a different child. The mother was slightly in shock. After all, she thought her baby had a 'problem', when all she needed to do was to make sure *she* was comfortable and relaxed and the 'problem' seemed to disappear.

In the following weeks she attended to her own level of tension, made sure she was comfortable when she interacted with her baby, and the baby gradually relaxed too – the power of body language.

How to get comfortable

• Get into the habit of noticing your physical position when you settle down with your baby for a feed or a cuddle. How do your shoulders feel? Do you have adequate support for elbows and head, so that your muscles can rest while you feed? Do you have items you may need close to hand? Would lying down be more in keeping with your needs than sitting? If you choose to lie down to feed your baby, make sure that you lie on the floor or on your bed rather than a sofa. Sofas are one of the danger spots in terms of co-sleeping because if you roll or your baby slides off you as you doze they can become trapped between your body and the back of the sofa or between the cushions and have problems breathing.

- Set up a couple of 'go-to' places in the house with the essentials to make you comfortable when you are feeding or cuddling: various cushions to prop your elbows and back, drinks and snacks, blankets in case you feel cold, a cosy rug to lie on if you prefer the floor to the bed in the daytime, books, magazines, remote controls if needed. Use these places as often as possible. If you have perineal discomfort it is often easier to recline or lie down when feeding, but if you want to sit up you can use a rubber ring or a long breastfeeding pillow arranged like a horseshoe beneath you to relieve the pressure on your perineum.

- If you are in physical pain postnatally, relieve it as best you can. Your midwife can help. If breastfeeding is causing any physical pain make sure you get support: this could be from your midwife or health visitor, a local breastfeeding group or by contacting a breastfeeding counsellor on one of the national helplines. A private lactation consultant (IBCLC) can help with complex problems and can carry out home visits. It is well worth sorting things out as fast as possible as being in pain creates tension, prevents the baby from feeding successfully and creates an even unhappier baby and mum – another of those spirals of discontent. The earlier you break that cycle the better! If the first person you ask can't help, keep trying until you find someone with the expertise you need.

The biggest surprise I had on becoming a mother was the amount of time I had to have my baby attached to my body. Whether on my breast or simply in my arms, some

*days it felt constant. I think it was a major contributor
to me starting to do all the cooking in the house. My
partner would come home and I would hand over the
baby, go cook dinner and rejoice in having the freedom to
move my body again. We went from sharing the cooking
to 'traditional' stereotypes all because of one baby!*

Your newborn is used to being 'held' by the muscular
uterine walls, so the freedom of life outside can come
as a bit of a shock. While it is important that babies do
not spend all their time wrapped and bundled, as they
need to have space to move their arms and legs freely,
it is something that you usually need to introduce
gradually. Here are some things you can try to avoid
overwhelming your baby in those early days and
weeks. (For video examples go to **www.pinterandmartin.
com/understanding-babies**).

- If your baby startles when you pass him to another
  person, you can make that transition a little easier
  by keeping your body in contact with your baby
  as long as possible as you pass him over, so that he
  has a near seamless experience of support rather
  than one of floating in space in your outstretched
  arms. You need to get very close to the person you
  are passing your baby to and take the transfer nice
  and slow. You will find the way that works in your
  particular situation: bending or sitting down to take
  the baby from your seated partner, or standing close
  and pausing a while with both of you in contact as
  you pass him between you.

- When changing his nappy either wrap a blanket quite firmly around his upper body with his arms bent up towards his face, or simply fold the lower half of his vest or babygro up around the arms to constrict them, giving him a sense of a boundary in one area while his legs are free in space.

- Swaddling your baby can make it easier for him to settle to sleep. If your baby only seems to be able to sleep on you and wakes whenever you try to put him down, it is something that you could try. You can swaddle a baby with hands constrained or with arms flexed and wrapped in close to the face. The advantage of the 'elbows bent' method is that your baby will be able to self-soothe by sucking on his fingers if necessary.

- However lovely holding your baby feels, there are also times when it is too much to bear: either you feel trapped or you actually need to do something else with your arms! It is easy to overlook the fact that there is more to your body than your arms and chest. If you are comfortable sitting cross-legged then placing your baby in your lap, cradled in your lap or with their belly on your thigh, can be a super quick alternative to give you a break.

- Babywearing is a wonderful way to keep both of you happy and content. When your baby is supported on your body, belly-to-belly, he feels your heart, smells your smell and with the combined constriction of the wrap and your movements experiences a sense of familiarity from his time in utero. There are many different types of wraps and slings on the market and it is important to choose one that feels comfortable for you: one size/style does *not* fit all. Professional advice and trying out the styles for fit and ease is important, and some shops offer this service; many areas also have 'sling libraries' where you can try out a variety of slings and wraps and take them home to really see how they suit you and your baby. There are also professional babywearing consultants who will do a home visit and bring a variety of wraps for you to try. It is vital that the sling or wrap you choose is suitable for a newborn baby: support for your baby's head and their hip positioning are super important. Professional fitting will ensure that both you and your baby are comfortable and safe. Also consider anyone else who will be baby wearing – they may need a different style of wrap or a different adjustment. For more information see *Why Babywearing Matters* by Rosie Knowles, also published by Pinter & Martin.

The art of giving and receiving touch

Mara and I had taken a nap on the rug together, through my dozing state I noticed she had started to make that grumbling sound that so often ended up with her crying. I put my hand on her belly, just lightly, thinking she was wanting to feel my presence near her. She paused but soon continued squirming and wiggling. I focussed on what I was feeling with my hand: her belly felt tight and hard. I made my touch even lighter, inviting her tummy to relax into the imaginary space I had created. I felt her start to relax; it was like her belly had expanded to fill the gap. It felt warm and I let my hand move lightly around with the movement of her belly. Mara calmed down, her movements subsided, she drifted back into sleep. Once I could feel she was peaceful I slowly moved my hand away and got a bit more sleep myself – it was amazing!

Touch in its most simple form is powerful. In somatic bodywork we use a light, receptive touch to 'listen' to the body and support a particular area or structure with our awareness. It may sound very esoteric, but it is something we all do when we feel discomfort: our instinct is to touch that place. Sometimes simply noticing the discomfort in this way will make the sensation change, and sometimes we might make our touch more active, and massage or rub the area so it feels better. Somatic bodyworkers are trained in attentiveness and anatomical/physiological knowledge over many years, but the skill of supporting another person through touch is something that we all possess.

Listening with your hand

Have a go to see what I mean. Just place your hand somewhere on your own torso, perhaps your belly or in the centre of your chest above the heart and lungs, and then make the touch really light – as if you were trying to touch the water standing in a bowl without disturbing the surface. Relax your hand and bring your attention to what you can feel happening underneath it. Close your eyes to help you focus and spend a few minutes allowing the sensations to come into your awareness. With practice you can feel not just the action of the breath moving the body, but also the organs moving within, the heart beating or the stomach churning. A warmth develops underneath your hand and if you are relaxed you will feel the area relax in response. You may feel like moving your hand gently with the sensation: follow your intuition! We are in the realm of the body and instinct is its language. When you give this kind of attentiveness to another person it can feel incredibly supportive.

There will be times when you look after your newborn when he is uncomfortable for a reason that you can't change. For example, many newborns complain when their tummy is digesting food or after a poo, due to the effort of the push and the sudden empty feeling when it's out. At times like this a simple hand on the abdomen can be soothing and support him to manage his emotion. You can also use it as a way to signal transitions and changes that your baby is about to experience, as explained in Chapter 1, and it can help settle your baby when they are restless.

Massage

The ancient art of baby massage spans many cultures, from Chinese Tui Na practice to the Ayurvedic traditions of India. While baby massage courses are quite easy to find, the nature of a group class makes them more suitable for older babies who are familiar with themselves and the world and less likely to be overwhelmed. And yet newborns can benefit enormously from massage too. It helps to stimulate digestion and balance hormonal activity, it offers the baby a sensory experience of their own body, and it aids bonding by helping parents tune into their baby's responses and expressions, likes and dislikes.

If your baby is very 'sleepy' in the first weeks, a massage can help ease him into the world. Rubbing the feet and using your fingers to press the soles of his feet in a gentle pulsing rhythm can support the action of suckling if he is finding suckling too effortful.

At the other end of the spectrum, a very sensitive and easily startled baby can benefit from a slow and rhythmic massage to bring him into a more relaxed state. Lots of belly-to-chest contact while carried in a wrap or sling is also calming and beneficial. If your baby finds massage too much at first, start with the listening touch as described above.

In the first couple of months, massage is usually performed in 'bits': a new baby will only tolerate massage for perhaps five minutes or so at one time (remember how tuned into touch and sensation they are – it is a lot to take in). He may also prefer to be held in your arms as you massage rather than lying in front of you. Just getting him used to being stroked is important and worth doing until he gets more comfortable with space around him. One idea is to link a particular massage stroke with a particular activity or time of day, so tummy strokes after changing nappies, or stroking the sides of the body while feeding. This little and often 'routine' means you don't forget to do it and your baby will get the full benefit.

Once your baby is happy to lie on a surface in front of you, you can combine a few massage strokes at a time, perhaps aiming for five to ten minutes at a time. If your baby is naked be aware that they may well relax enough to wee! So if you have a son, I would advise you to lie a bit of a towel or cloth lightly on top of his penis, so that you don't end up with a fountain in your face (you have been warned!). If your baby is happy to be naked or partially naked, use a vegetable-based baby massage oil. You may want to avoid scented oils for the first few weeks, in which case organic rapeseed oil is a cheap and easy-to-find alternative.

By the time your baby is nearing three months old, you will probably be able to massage your baby on a changing mat and may wish to start introducing some routines into your baby's day, so think about when a massage would be most useful. If massage tends to wake up or excite your baby make it part of your morning playtime, but if you find he relaxes with it, use it later in the day when you both need a break, or in the evening prior to the final feed of the day. Now is a great time to do a baby massage course if you are feeling the need to meet other people who are caring for little ones.

The key to a good massage is – yes, I'll say it again – your own level of relaxation and responsiveness. So make sure your hands and arms are relaxed, perhaps by putting on a bit of nice, flowing music and doing a little hand and arm dance to shake or roll out any tension before you start. You can massage your baby according to a specific technique or simply intuitively: the main thing to focus on is to keep your fingers or hand in constant contact with the skin as you stroke. If your touch is so light that the fingers skip over the skin it becomes ticklish and will overwhelm your baby's nervous system in a way that will make them tense up. Be confident to offer your baby a little more pressure with your stroke, in particular on the upper arms and legs where the bigger muscles are. Think of the massage as a dialogue: watch your baby's reactions, go slow and give him time to respond to let you know if he is enjoying the experience. Your hands can tell you a lot too: notice if he is relaxed or tense, if he moves towards or away from your touch or if he becomes more or less alert as you repeat a particular stroke. Get to know your baby's body language.

Simple massage suggestions

When your baby is cradled in your arm, work on the side furthest away from your body.

- Stroke down from the shoulder to the hand, allowing your thumb to gently press your baby's palm so that he reflexively grasps your finger. Then, when he is holding on to your thumb, very gently mobilise the joint by jiggling it softly and move the whole arm from the shoulder joint in a slow, gentle arm dance.

- Long strokes from under the arm along the body and down the leg to the foot.

- Rubbing the sole of the foot. A lovely stroke from the Tui Na tradition is 'Kneading the Gushing Spring'. This is great for calming your baby and helping him fall asleep. Press your finger or thumb into the centre of the ball of the foot (two-thirds along the midline from the back of the heel to the base of the toe), make a circular kneading motion fifty times, then from that point, stroke up to the base of the toes fifty times.

With baby in front of you or in your arms.
To aid digestion and elimination (if baby has wind the massage will move it through his intestines so he might seem a bit more uncomfortable before he lets it out and feels happy again.)

- Massage clockwise (as you are looking at your baby) with three fingers directly round the belly button.

- Hold your baby's feet with the soles together so the hips fall open to the sides and circle the legs over his belly clockwise.

Starfish massage
From about six to eight weeks of age, or once your baby is less curled up, you can add the starfish massage stroke, which follows the radial symmetry of your baby's nervous system and supports their growing awareness of their own body.

- With your baby lying on his back, rest both hands lightly on his navel.

- Starting when your hands rise in response to an in breath, move both your hands simultaneously up and out along both arms to your baby's palms and then back to centre. Repeat, maintaining a slow, steady rhythm, 8–10 times or as long as enjoyed. Try and synchronise the movement out from the navel with an in breath, but then allow the stroke to last several of your baby's breath cycles.

- Repeat, but this time moving the hands down along the legs to the feet and back to the centre. Slow, steady, 8–10 times, always starting at the navel.

- In the same way, starting from the navel each time, explore different combinations of limbs; right leg and arm, right arm and left leg, both arms, both legs, and so on.

This massage stroke can also be performed with your baby lying on his tummy, head turned to the side and resting on the mat. You start the stroke from the approximate place of the navel from behind, at the top of the sacrum. When working on the back you can include the head and the bottom of the spine as two 'limbs' and move your hands from the centre up and down the spine, then back to centre, as you do with the limbs, then explore the combinations of arms, legs, head and 'tail' (bottom of the spine).

Texture massage

By the end of the first three months, when your baby starts to be interested in playing with their hands and feet, you can use massage to support sensory nerve maturation with the texture massage game. Select some interesting textures for him to feel with his hands and bare feet. You can use anything you have to hand: fabric, clean stones, any kind of brush, a feather, your breath, your lips. Take things very slowly and give your baby a bit of time in between textures to respond and register the sensations he is feeling.

When touch seems to be unwelcome

We don't expect our babies to wriggle, complain and arch away from us whenever we hold them close. But some children do just that, consistently. It can be really distressing for parents and in the heady weeks of hormone shifts that follow the birth, parents can feel very rejected, and as if they are somehow failing when their baby behaves this way. The conventional approach is to simply respect your baby's preference and, rather than sit and cuddle, increase the time you spend face to face with them, having little 'play conversations', talking together, mirroring your baby and so forth. While this is a useful strategy to help you bond with and feel closer to your baby, you run the risk of overwhelming them with stimulation, as we have already discussed. So it is important to look behind the behaviour to try to uncover the reason for it, and seek professional help if you wish.

While you are deciding what to do, I would advise you to maintain lots of body-to-body contact with your child, in the most sensitive way possible. If the problem for your baby is being held constricted in your arms, then place them in your lap while you sit cross-legged, or lie down with them lying on your belly, or simply next to you physically touching. If feeding in your arms is difficult, try lying down to feed instead. If your baby has a high tone (they may hold themselves stiffly, or seem tense – see p111) but strategies like swaddling or babywearing just make him more upset, see if he will tolerate lying on his side, curled up with you next to him, or even lying on his belly (on your belly or on the floor): these positions can help reduce stimulation for your baby and help them relax. A baby hammock or using a blanket to rock your baby in can be helpful to give him a gentle contained feeling and relax body and senses.

Massage is also a good idea, if done sensitively. Focusing on the belly area, either with massage or just a listening hand, may help your baby settle, as well as the 'Kneading the Gushing Spring' technique. Notice the details: is it a particular part of the body that your child wants to have free from constraint? Is their head position balanced, or are they holding it to one side when lying horizontally? Is there a quality of touch that they are less unhappy with: light stroking, deep pressure, kissing? When you find something they tolerate, do it more. Your aim is to maintain some physical connection without adding to the stress your child experiences, so just try one thing a day, and if it seems to be accepted then repeat throughout the day, slowly and with confidence, rather than trepidation, although I know that can be a tall order. As always, how you feel in your body – relaxed, confident or otherwise – will transmit to your baby.

If you decide to seek professional support, your options always include your doctor, midwife or health visitor, or someone like a craniosacral therapist, osteopath or bodyworker who is specially trained to work with babies.

3

MOVEMENT IS KEY

*Movement is singularly important as the exclusive
language of the first year of life and remains central to
communication throughout life...*

Ruella Frank and Frances La Barre,
The First Year and the Rest of your Life

We have looked at how your baby needs your help to
regulate her emotions and acclimatise to life on the
'outside', discussed the developmental significance
of touch, both physically and emotionally, and now
we come to the last and most misunderstood of the
three development fundamentals: movement. A whole
chapter on movement for a baby that cannot even hold
their head up independently? Yes, that's right, because
movement is not just about gross and fine motor skills
or even muscular strength; it is integral to all aspects of
our development: physical, intellectual and emotional.

Our movement organises and integrates the whole of the central nervous system. It influences learning and expression, how we experience and interact with the world around us, emotion, learning skills and actions. When you support natural movement development you are nurturing your baby's intellectual and emotional development, not just her physicality. Complex and nuanced as the information in this chapter may seem at first, if you follow the physical explorations you will soon see the practical applications. We will be talking about what to offer your child in terms of physical experience when you hold her, feed her, and how she might spend her time when she is not in your arms. All these everyday interactions have the potential to support your child or make things a little more difficult for her. To be able to balance your needs and hers, you need to understand what is important and why. Then you can be confident and creative with the choices you make. Knowledge is power!

Movement development

If you look up baby movement development online or in a book, you will most likely find it explained in terms of movement milestones that you should expect your baby to master by specific ages. Babies learn to roll, then crawl (on their belly and later on their hands and knees), and once they are crawling on hands and knees they can sit independently and kneel, stand, cruise the furniture and eventually walk unsupported. The focus is mostly on the age by which each skill is to be mastered rather than understanding how the different milestones express and develop your baby's abilities, and this can create a lot of misunderstanding. Parents assume that faster is better. They watch their child anxiously, comparing their progress with other babies, and worry if they don't develop in a linear fashion. Some will buy products like baby walkers, or try to train their baby's abdominals by pulling them into sit-ups in order to speed up the process. Not only are these practices unnecessary, they will make life harder for your child. While there is an organic time frame within which each pattern emerges, the speed with which your baby acquires movement skills does not indicate her level of intelligence or her ability to succeed in life. I've checked it out and the studies that have explored these questions pretty much cancel each other out in their findings. I suspect they may have been asking the wrong question, and here's why.

The journey of movement development is in essence circuitous. Rather than climbing up a mountain of achievements, your baby will spend this next year wandering up and down a hilly neighbourhood. Your baby might spend a few days in total frustration as she tries to roll and then when she works it out, spend the next few weeks contentedly lying on her back and playing with her hands and feet as if she has forgotten that rolling was even possible. Then one day she will start rolling again as if it is second nature. She may spend weeks rolling right round the room to get to places, she may simply roll to her belly and start pushing between hands and feet to try move up to all fours, or explore rolling in some other way entirely of her own choosing. Each journey is individual, and our full experience of each pattern is affected by our environment, our physique, how our parents interact with us, our preferences and our particular needs. Movement must be functional, and to that end we need to be flexible and adaptable in the way we move. Within each milestone or pattern we need to find balance, and align our bodies, our intention and perception in a way that is adaptable to different circumstances. To learn that flexibility we need a wide variety of experiences and challenges. As we progress through the first year we dip in and out of different patterns of movements on different planes in space, weaving an intricate web of form and function that creates connections within the brain to achieve maximum function for minimum effort both physically and mentally.

Let's take an example you can relate to and track just a tiny part of your newborn's movement repertoire. In the first weeks you may notice how your baby wriggles, the impulse starting from the coccyx or 'tail' of her spine. That impulse will initiate the rolling movements she starts to make a few months down the line. Later still that same roll, again initiated from the tail but this time with her body up on its hands and knees, will help her shift her body back down from crawling to sitting and help her twist her body from side to side, ready to interact with people and things. In fact that rolling motion is also teaching her eyes to track objects while they move and underlies her ability to track the words on the pages as she reads a book in the future. When you realise how much each movement pattern is teaching us, you will perhaps understand why we tend to take a very individual route through the overall sequence.

If we are also mindful of what we know about how the brain develops, I think it is fair to speculate that it is the *variety* of movement exploration that could potentially make a difference to a child's intellectual and emotional capacities, rather than the speed at which skills are mastered. As we have already seen, our brains build neurological connections in response to our experiences: each variation creates a new connection. The more varied the experiences your baby gathers, the greater the number of neurological connections her brain has to choose from when it prunes through the structures and decides on the most efficient and effective ones for her to use. So you can see that the time your baby takes to explore the various movements she can make is time well spent. Experimenting with which part of her body initiates action, how it feels to move on different surfaces, from different starting positions, and the quality of the movements themselves, all add to the richness of her learning. Working it out for herself will give her a sense of achievement and build self-confidence rather than dependency.

If you speed your baby along, constantly encouraging her to move one step further, or place her in positions she cannot attain by herself, you will inevitably create emotional stress by putting her in situations that she has not yet got the capacity to regulate for herself. If your newborn is constantly held vertical, facing outwards to the world in a sling, for example, how difficult are you making it for her to pace her level of excitement? It is much easier to shut out the world and relax your face on your parent's chest than to close your eyes and rest when everything is there, right in front of you. A parent may choose to carry their child that way because it seems to calm them, which it may in the short term, but not in a restful way – it is hyper-stimulation, and that will build throughout the day and in the long term it can affect your baby's level of contentment, or the quality of their sleep and yours. Over time, you may find that your child demands constant entertainment (that level of arousal that we talked about in Chapter 1 is set high). A few months on and that same baby might find it boring to lie on her tummy, and that will mean that getting up to crawling takes longer than she wants it to, and that frustration will affect many aspects of your life. It is an imaginary trajectory, but can you see how a very small, seemingly insignificant decision – carrying your baby facing outwards – can spiral into something with a huge impact on your baby and your family. At any point in that imaginary trajectory above, parents can adjust their way of caring for their baby, but the later that happens the more difficult it can be and the more effort it requires, which is why awareness and knowledge are so important.

While the journey itself, in the case of development at least, is more significant than the arrival at your destination, there are parameters. If your baby is very delayed in acquiring a movement skill even though she is in a supportive environment it can indicate underlying neurological difficulties and in some countries regular developmental checks are carried out by doctors to ensure early intervention where needed. Like most things, the earlier you deal with it the easier it is to sort out, and this can take the form of physiotherapy or movement education sessions. This is why a good understanding of how movement development works is so important for parents: not only does it prevent anxiety and ensure you can confidently support your child, but it will also help you perceive and therefore address any difficulties that may arise promptly. We will discuss what you should be aware of as we go through the movements in detail later in the chapter, but let's start at the very beginning and look at how we move into life.

The developmental movement sequence

The developmental movement sequence starts organising our body before we are even born. Your baby starts moving inside you as soon as she has grown her arms and legs. From about 56 days after conception she reflexively curls and uncurls her limbs, flexes and extends the spine and orientates her movements around the umbilical cord. She explores moving different combinations of limbs and spine in a pattern of radial symmetry called 'navel radiation'. As she matures, her movements become larger and more purposeful: your baby somersaults, stretches, pushes and bounces. Movements also become finer and more precise: your baby explores with fingers and toes, touching and finding her mouth and face, hands playing, feet pressing and feeling the resistance of the womb, all within the supportive fluid environment of the amniotic sac.

The sensations your baby experiences within your body, the constant massage of your heart and lungs, the periodic churning of your stomach and intestines, the variety of positions and movements you make every day, are registered by her vestibular system and used to help build new neural connections within her brain. The vestibular system, which regulates balance and spatial awareness, is the very first sensory system to mature. At birth it is better developed than hearing, smell and eyesight. It is located within the structure of the ear and it helps your baby orient herself to gravity, before she has even realised where her own body ends and the world begins.

During the birth process your baby's ability to fold and unfold, curl and stretch her whole body will help her respond to the pressure of your uterine muscles and find her way down and out. She will push and wiggle within your pelvis and her head will reach and rotate as she journeys out into the world. As she travels through the birth canal she will experience her first full stretch for months. It is slow, rhythmical and strong; stimulating the body, activating hormonal and cardiovascular systems, and then, suddenly, it is over. Your baby enters an unfamiliar world, and curls right up again. It will take several weeks for her to lengthen into her fullness and curling up close in your arms will help her feel calm and safe until she is ready to do so.

As tender and vulnerable as your newborn baby

seems as she wiggles and jerks her body in the unfamiliar air-filled environment, her reflexes are primed to aid her survival. If placed naked, tummy down on mum's belly, she can crawl up to find and latch on to the breast for her first feed. If you press your finger into your newborn's palm, she will grasp it tightly, and if she is startled she will stretch and open her whole body in distress in the Moro reflex, before curling up again, fingers grasping for something to hold on to, finding her calm by moving her body into that familiar flexed position. The rooting and suckling reflex that your baby has been practising for many months means she can search for your nipple, reaching with her mouth, and when she finds it she can open wide, latch on and feed.

Over the next few months your baby will practise all the movements from the womb without the support of the amniotic fluid. You will be able to watch the navel radiation pattern, supporting her to move arms and legs as well enabling her to curl in and stretch out her whole body. She will wiggle and wriggle her spine and over time keep her head in line with her spine without the extra support of your hand. You may find that she even wriggles away from you when you place her on her back or tummy on a firm surface. While a lot of focus is put on muscle development and having a strong neck, you might be surprised that it is her ability to relax and relate to gravity with a yield that will help her get moving, rather than any tendency to hold tension. You can prove that yourself: try lying down on your side on the floor, tense your whole body and roll to your belly... and now try yielding your weight into the floor to roll from side to belly and back, letting your breath flow with your movement. Which felt more effortful, which was more comfortable?

As she reaches the three-month mark you will probably see your baby's movements start to organise in different ways, with a homologous symmetry developing where both arms do the same thing and both legs do something different to the arms. For example, her hands may be clasped in front of her chest while she bashes both heels into the floor as she lies on her back. Soon she will be playing with hands and feet, clasping her hands together as she lies on her back, in line with the midline of her body that runs in the same direction as her spine. It will take a few more weeks for her to start reaching across it. As she lies on her back she will endlessly practise reaching for toys, toes or fingers, accurately measuring distance, calibrating thrust, angle of approach and control of her limbs so that she can grab and hold on to what interests her. When she lies on her belly she will support her weight on her forearms and look at the world from this new perspective.

By four months of age, your baby may already have started to show an interest in rolling from the back to the front of her body. She may be making an effort to roll, or she may find it by accident. Noticing these qualities and her response to the event will tell you a bit more about her personality. Mastering the roll over the next few months will enable her to decide for herself if she wants to play on her back or her belly. Playing on her tummy will enable her to find the floor with her big toe and start to explore the 'just out of reach' environment by belly crawling (a homolateral, left side/right side organisation of the body). Eventually she will learn how to come up to crawling on hands and knees and move with a contralateral symmetry, right arm, left leg then left arm right leg. And so, having mastered the patterns, she is free to spiral her body in and out of sitting, pull herself up to standing, walk, hop, then skip and jump through the rest of her childhood and beyond!

Exploring movement patterns

Reading about the patterns you will see her explore in the next three to four months is not going to give you the full picture. You need to find them and experience them yourself: after all, they were instrumental in your own development, so it is really a kind of remembering. I would recommend exploring one pattern at a time, by reading the section, then doing the exploration. If your baby is already here, spend a bit of time observing them to check out what they are doing and then have another go. This way you give your body time to integrate the information. Once you have explored all the patterns you can try to work out how to sequence from one to the next, to understand how each pattern supports the subsequent one.

While it may feel a bit strange moving 'like a baby', your body will appreciate the chance to revisit these fundamental patterns. If you take the time to relax into the exercises you will come away refreshed, with new information about your own body as well as your baby. Indeed, somatic practitioners often work with developmental patterns with adults when dealing with chronic physical or psychological issues. It is never too late to repattern our neurology! So get down on a blanket and join me. Tempting as it may be to simply read the texts, the MP3s which you can access at **www. pinterandmartin.com/understanding-babies** will make this part of the book easier to follow.

I promise you that doing the explorations is going to give you so much more than just reading about them.

Navel radiation

Have you ever seen a video of a starfish moving underwater? All the starry limbs seem to be controlled from its central point, furling and unfurling in a wave-like motion. That pattern of motion underlies our movement as soon as we have created our bodies. We call it navel radiation and you can observe it in utero on 4D scans when babies focus their movement around the umbilicus or navel. This energetic connection extends out from the navel along each limb and to the top and bottom of the spine. Bringing support from the centre to the extremities of the body is our first pattern of organisation. When you do the exploration, pay attention to your sensory and emotional experience.

Exercise: Starfish adult exploration

You can do this exploration in any position, but it is particularly nice to start lying curled up on your side with your eyes closed. As you come into movement you will find yourself rolling onto your back.

Make sure you are lying down comfortably. Take a moment to notice how you feel physically and emotionally. Let your mind settle...

Focus your awareness on your belly, your navel – notice how it moves out and in with each breath you take.

Imagine that the air is coming into your body through your navel. Feel it filling up your ribcage. Can you feel how your shoulders respond to the in breath, widening, releasing?

Picture the air flowing from your navel up through your shoulders and along your arms to the very tips of your fingers. Breathe through that connection from tummy to fingertips.

Imagine that the air is coming into your body through your navel. Feel it filling up your pelvis, notice how your hips respond to the in breath with a slight turn out, and back again as you breathe out.

Picture the air flowing from your navel and down through your legs to the toes. Breathe along that connection.

Imagine that the air is coming into your body through your navel and feel it filling up your spinal column. Sense the way your spine reaches up at your head, and down with its tail as you breathe in and how it relaxes, subtly curling forward towards your navel at both ends when you breathe out.

Notice the way your limbs, your head and your tail respond to the breath.

Allow the breath to carry your limbs into movement. Let them move in and out from your navel, gently and slowly floating on your breath...

Keep elbows and knees gently folding and soft, move slowly.

Feel the connection to the navel and let your whole body respond and change position as you explore.

Notice how it feels to be opened out, how it feels to curl up.

Explore moving different combinations of limbs... folding and unfolding. Head and legs – feel the connection down to your toes. One arm and one leg – explore other combinations and let them move your body as much as you feel like today.

Let the breath and your connection through the navel support your movement.

As you move allow your breath to energise your body. Feel every cell filling with fresh air and energy.

When you are ready to finish, slowly allow your

eyes to open. Notice how your body feels now. Is the experience complete? Do you need to stretch or move or change position? Do you feel any different from when you started? How?

Now that you have felt that navel connection that underlies your newborn's movements, you will be better able to see it. At first the movements might seem jerky: she is used to being supported by fluid, but as she practises her movements will become smoother and vary in speed and energy. As she gains the ability to move more smoothly you might notice that when she is overstimulated she loses it and her movements become more jerky again – a sign to take note of and act upon by reducing stimulation. By the end of three months she will be able to really stretch and flex her body, reaching with her head or tail or even with her belly button. At first though, her torso may seem relatively still and simply initiate the movement of her limbs.

Did you notice any emotional response to being curled up versus stretched out? Being able to curl up and turn your focus inward when things are getting too much is a basic survival strategy that the navel radiation pattern makes possible. It is in essence our first 'yes', when moving towards, and our first 'no', when withdrawing. You may have noticed how the movement relates to the Moro or startle reflex, which happens when your baby is surprised or her head moves out of line with her spine. In the Moro she will cry and jerk her body backwards, with arms, legs, mouth and eyes wide open. Guiding her into the second phase of this reflex, a curled up position, with legs and arms bent, secure in your arms after such a 'startle response', will help her to regulate her emotions.

Spinal patterns

The first spinal movements happen in utero as part of the flexion and extension of the spine that supports your baby's birth. Your baby's spine is soft, flexible and shaped in a C. She has yet to develop the cervical (neck) and lumbar (lower back) curves that will ensure she can maintain a vertical position easily. The muscles and connective tissues have to learn to share the effort of maintaining stability, yet allow flexibility. This job is most efficiently done starting from a horizontal position and experiencing gravity through the front and back surfaces of your body in equal measure. The cervical curve develops as your baby learns to support the weight of her head away from gravity and her lumbar curve will develop as she starts to crawl and walk.

Spinal patterns explore sequencing and direction. Your baby will move her spine sequentially when she lies on the front, back or side of her body – rather like an inchworm. She will initiate the movement from her head, and over time start to initiate also from the bottom of her spine or 'tail'. This clear initiation from top or bottom helps her later to direct her body through space as she crawls or moves vertically into sitting.

Adults' spines are notorious for feeling tense or blocked in certain areas; chronic tension is not uncommon.

Pregnancy postural changes, with the addition of the postnatal carrying and cuddling of a young baby, can make your back and shoulders achy and uncomfortable. Try this gentle spinal exploration to look after your spine as well as give you some insight into your baby's movement. It is very easy to do with a wakeful baby: simply lie your baby on the floor and position yourself on all fours above her so you are face-to-face. This way, if she wants your attention you are right there to play. If your wrists are uncomfortable in this position you can rest your body weight on your forearms, but you may need to put cushions under your arms to make sure there is space for your baby if she is going to be with you.

Exercise: Spinal adult exploration

Based on the Cat (Marjaryasana) *and Cow* (Bitilasana) *yoga asanas.*

Start kneeling.

Take a moment to simply touch your spine – the bits you can easily reach with your arms. Notice how your spine feels. Are there any areas of tension? Now let your head and hands reach forward and bring your body into all fours.

Release your toes so the front surfaces of your feet and toes are in contact with the floor. If this feels uncomfortable you can place a rolled-up towel under the front of your feet to let them relax more easily.

Just breathe.

See if you can notice the slight expansion of your spine on the in breath.

Now notice the reverse action on the out breath. Your spine subtly curls forward and down at both ends.

When you have found that feeling in your body, imagine your breath flowing into your spine through your navel and expanding it as you breathe in – head and tail moving towards the sky.

When you breathe out again, let your spine arch (like a cat) so that your head and tail move down to the floor and your navel moves up and away from it.

Start the movements small and gentle and let your breath massage your spine awake. Keep your elbows slightly bent, soft and mobile as you alternate between the two positions with your breath.

Breathe in to reach head and tail up to the ceiling. Breathe out to reach them down to the floor.

Picture a soft, flexible, fluid spine moving with the support of your breath.

Now start to explore the space with your spine. Let it move in all directions, softly twisting and swinging as it wishes.

Experiment by leading the movement with the head end and see how it sequences through. Now initiate movement from the tail end of your spine.

How does that feel?

Keep hands/forearms and knees planted on the floor but elbows soft, so that the rest of the body can respond to your spinal movements.

Alternate speed and pace.

When you feel ready, allow your spine to bring you up to sitting or kneeling. Notice how it feels – is there a difference?

The spinal exploration can be very energising in a relaxed way. It supports your abdominal muscles and pelvic floor (when initiating movement from the tail or coccyx), increasing blood flow to the area to promote healing and gently activating the muscles.

The exercise will also give you a sense of what moving from the spine feels like. There is a condensing of the very core of your body and an inner coherence that comes with these movements. The sequencing through from head to tail organises the body's direction in space, so reaching from either end expresses a desire to move forward or back.

Towards the end of the third month you may start to see your baby adding homologous movements (see below) to her repertoire. Our exploration combines both homologous movements and rolling, which most babies start to experiment with at some time during the fourth or fifth month.

Homologous movements

Homologous movement describes a symmetry between the top and bottom half of the body. So any movement where both legs are doing the same thing, or both arms are doing the same thing, is a homologous movement. You will see these movements start to happen towards the end of the first three months, when your baby starts clasping her hands together and bringing them to her mouth, or holding them above her chest in the midline. She may start flexing her knees with her legs suspended above her body and perhaps reaching for them with her hands. When she lies on her belly your baby will be able to support her upper body with both forearms pressed into the floor. Homologous movement becomes even more prominent over the next three months as your baby becomes more comfortable with playing on her belly and starts to explore pushing up out of gravity with hands, knees and feet, as well as reaching out to space in the airplane position.

Rolling

The movement milestone of rolling is just around the corner for your three-month-old baby. Usually it happens when your baby is playing happily on her back, legs and arms moving above her body, perhaps playing with a toy, and your baby quite suddenly finds herself lying on her side. The weight and the momentum of her arms and legs have simply acquiesced to gravity and pulled her body over. If she is relaxed she may have enough momentum to roll right over on to her belly. Our first roll happens in one piece: the whole spine rotates, taking our torso with it, and when we come to our belly both arms (once they are available – one has a habit of getting stuck underneath) will help raise the chest off the floor by pushing into the floor to take weight on to the forearms.

Exercise: Symmetry and rolling adult exploration

If you are doing this later in pregnancy, follow your midwife / doctor's advice about lying on your back, and only go as far as rolling from side to side. Lying on your back for an extended time may make you feel dizzy, as your uterus can compress major veins and arteries.

Lie on your back next to your baby with knees bent and feet on the floor. Take a moment just to breathe and relax your back and head on the floor.

Now lift your arms so that your fingers meet above your body at your midline. Touch your fingers together and start to stroke, massage and explore your hands and arms. Be aware of the physical sensation of your touch. Vary its pace... its quality... its purpose. Notice the shapes your fingers and arms make as they move.

When you are ready, let your right hand rest on your right shoulder, left hand on the left shoulder and simultaneously slowly stroke down both sides of your body and along your thighs until you approach your knees.

Lift your feet off the floor and continue to explore your legs and your feet if you can reach them comfortably with your hands.

Now rest your arms and let your feet explore each other in the air. Notice how your legs turn out in the hip joint as your feet meet at the midline of your body.

Let your arms and legs float in the air above you. You might try out some homologous movement here, doing the same action with both arms or with both legs at once... how does it make you feel?

When you are ready to roll, with legs and arms bent, let the leg and arm on the side you wish to roll to slowly fall to that side and bring the opposite arm and leg with it so that your spine rolls in one piece, like a log, to the side.

Explore rolling from one side to the other, and if you want to, allow the roll to take you on to your front. Find the easiest, least effortful way to roll.

Notice how being relaxed makes the roll easy and more comfortable than if your body is either tensed with effort or totally collapsed into the floor. Try out both extremes, tense and collapsed, and find a comfortably relaxed middle way.

Explore rolling. Is going to one side easier than going to the other? If so, why?

You can finish here, resting on your side and slowly pushing up to sitting when ready, or if you are able to, continue on to your belly.

Roll on to your belly, with elbows bent at about shoulder level. Breathe in deeply and notice how your lungs fill with air and start to lift your chest away from the floor.

Relax on your front with your head turned to one side. Allow your body to feel the support of the floor, then yield your weight to gravity. Can you sense a moment where it feels right to push away from the floor again?

Take some time to find this subtle rebound from the floor, then use it to press down with your forearms and bring your chest away from the floor as far as is comfortable.

Ride this impulse a few more times, using a large in breath to support you up. Notice what it feels like to be at this level of perception.

Find a relaxed way to roll back on to your side or your back and take a rest.

Notice how your body feels. How much effort did you use floating your arms and legs above you? Did you notice how the navel radiation pattern was supporting you? And with the pushing up onto your forearms and rolling, was it easier and more comfortable when you released your weight into the floor or when you tensed your body?

Movement requires effort, for sure, but it also requires a judicious use of our physical resources, not just a lot of muscle power. Bonnie Bainbridge Cohen identified four stages of effort that underlie our movements: yield, push, reach and pull. And it is that first term 'yield', the physical release into the support of gravity, that is key to having a comfortable and easy experience of moving.

Newton's third law of motion states that for every action there is an equal and opposite reaction. If we allow our weight to release into the floor, we will experience an equivalent rebound: it's small and subtle, but it is all that we need to initiate the push that can bring our body to another level or into motion. As adults we are so used to this yield that we don't notice it anymore. If you pay close attention when you stand up from a chair, for example, you will notice that your feet sink into the floor a little bit in order to support the push up with the leg muscles, and your head reaches and pulls the body forward through space to walk. The yield and push is followed by a reach and pull. In the same way, your baby yields to the pressure of the uterine muscles in order to then push away with her feet, then reach with her head to bring her body into the world.

In the rolling exploration above I emphasised yielding your weight into the ground to roll and letting the lungs support your ribcage to rise away from the floor, rather than tensing your back to pull yourself up. We don't often consider our organs as part of our movement, but they support us not just in their function, but also with their form. I hope you were able to perceive the difference in effort and comfort moving with different levels of yield/tension created in your body.

How to support natural movement development

Floor play

Your baby seeks safety and support. Bonding with your baby, that confirmation that you are there for them whatever, is a physical act as much as an emotional feeling. Your baby needs to be able to yield her weight into your body and to feel it is there and able to connect, support and sustain her. In the first few weeks this is the experience your baby will seek above any other. Once that physical bond is established and your baby starts to realise that her body is actually separate to yours, she needs to bond to the earth. This is when floor play needs to become a significant part of your daily routine.

Your comfortable presence down there with your child is key. That means you need the right amount of blankets, mats, futons, cushions, beanbags – whatever you need to feel relaxed and content so that your baby does too. Take the time you need to adjust, prop and basically make yourself feel heavenly. Your presence is vital, so start hanging out together on the floor as soon as you want to. It rather depends on how you both feel in terms of her need for swaddling and your own postnatal recovery. However, at some stage within the first two months, when your baby becomes more confident without swaddling, getting used to the floor as a place for playing and resting together is an important step. Apart from providing your baby with space to freely move, unrestricted by car seats and cuddles, joining her down on the floor will help her feel acknowledged and help you notice the detail of her movement language.

Meeting your baby at their own physical level of possibility rather than constantly bringing them up to yours may feel harder for you at the moment, but it is really worth making it a regular and substantial part of your day. Floor play is your baby's equivalent of going to the gym. The more time your baby spends here, the easier it will be for her to master the movement patterns and come up to vertical when she is ready. If your baby spends most of her time vertical, at 'adult' level, then she will want to stay where the action is, even when she is heavier and it is harder for you to sustain. Her expectations will not match her own abilities and that can result in a lot of frustration for you to deal with.

With variation in mind to support her learning, have some different textures for your baby to lie on. A firm surface like wood or linoleum flooring will make her spinal movements more successful in actually moving her body through space, for example. Make sure she can experience lying on her tummy and sides as well as her back. There is more detailed information about creating an enjoyable tummy playtime for your baby in the next chapter.

Once your baby is finding her feet, make sure she has sock-free time: we use our feet very sensitively to discover the world and master shifts of weight and pressure, even before we stand up on them. If cold feet are an issue, then get used to simply alternating socks on and socks off in five to ten minute intervals during play time, or cut the toes and heel off a pair of warm socks.

If your level of mobility makes it difficult to get down to the floor, you can give your baby a similar experience by placing her on a big table and sitting so that your face is at her level, which means you can maintain a close connection with her. Make sure you do not leave her unattended even for a moment. Big beds will offer her some variation in terms of her physical experience, as will textured blankets or materials on a higher surface for her to lie on. Face-to-face with a baby gives you an opportunity to play games, making faces or using rattles and toys to draw her interest.

Observing your baby's movement

Adults are so used to 'reading' other people's facial expressions and listening to their words that it can be hard to relate to a young baby whose face and vocalising are not yet under their conscious control. Watching the detail of their movements: where their effort is directed, how relaxed or excited they seem, whether they are moving towards or away from something, are all aspects of movement that can bring you additional information about a situation. Psychotherapists Ruella Frank and Frances La Barre add two additional movements to Bonnie Bainbridge Cohen's sequence, describing six fundamental movements of yield, push, reach, pull, grasp and release, which your baby will master as she moves through the developmental movement sequence to fulfil her physical and emotional needs.

These movements become part of the baby's efforts to self-regulate and regulate interpersonal relationships. They are essential to character development in that they become the preferred and routine ways we dynamically adjust, making them simultaneously psychological and physical by nature.[2]

Notice how long your three-month-old tries to manipulate a toy to bring the red wooden ring to her mouth. When she drops it, does she cry with frustration? Does she flap her arms and make a noise and try to get your attention to help? Is she still and resigned? Will she immediately turn her attention to something else or pause? Does her whole body tense up with anger and effort? What does this tell you about her forming personality? Do you recognise any of those responses as your own habitual responses? When she finally manages to grasp a toy, do you give her enough time to truly enjoy it before offering her another play idea, or do you interrupt her satisfaction? These are the kinds of questions you can ask yourself as you watch your baby play. You will get a feel for how she paces her learning, so that you respond in play more sensitively. Often the value of doing this is simply to help you feel more confident in your initial response: we read bodies unconsciously after all.

Attending to the physical

Paying attention to your baby's physical development can include noticing that they are struggling with something in particular. Appreciating your baby as they are is important, but there are two quite common issues that you might observe that can limit the choices they have and make things more difficult as they develop. Being aware of these issues means you can adapt your own behaviour to support your baby to find more ease as they move and grow.

The first relates to the ease with which your baby turns her head from left to right or vice versa. Most babies (and adults) have a preferred side – it feels easier to turn your head one way or the other. Try it! While your baby will not be able to support the weight of their head in vertical for some time, they are able turn their head side-to-side when lying on their back. So if you notice that they favour one side significantly, it is worth making an effort to play and relate to them from the side they don't particularly like. It's the everyday stuff – which side you approach them to lift them into your arms, how you carry them and those little games you play – just do it more on the less popular side. Often people find they are unconsciously supporting an imbalance because they prefer to hold or carry their baby in a particular way. The key here is to entice and encourage your baby to start looking to the other side, not to manipulate or force her head. If the issue persists it may indicate an alignment injury from their birth and it may be helpful to seek osteopathic or chiropractic help.

The second issue relates to your baby's ease of movement in general. You are probably used to hearing about tone in the context of the way your muscles look. However, your baby is born with an underlying tissue tone, a more global level of tension/relaxation within the body. When you explored rolling and collapsed your weight fully into the floor (low tone) it made it very difficult to move. The same is true when you tense your body (high tone) – you need even more energy to move when your body feels stiff. Of course we naturally move between these levels of tone, and different tasks require different levels of tension, but noticing if your baby's general, 'most of the time' tone leans to one extreme or the other can help you bring them into balance.

You may notice your baby has high tone if she startles easily, seems to have very 'advanced' head control, but is unwilling/unable to rest her head to the side when she lays on her belly. A high tone baby may have difficulties feeding and discomfort digesting. She will probably demand lots of cuddling and suckling opportunities. Suckling is her natural way to find a more balanced tone, her way of relaxing and connecting to the parasympathetic nervous system. High tone might be a result of a stressful pregnancy, birth or simply the level of anxiety, excitement or tension that your baby finds around her. Practices like babywearing and spending time lying on her belly in a relaxed and restful way will help your baby start to come to balance. Taking particular care not to overstimulate a high tone baby is also helpful, by protecting her inner awareness and making sure she has every opportunity to rest and nap.

At the opposite end of the scale is the low tone baby, a baby that is very sleepy and floppy, and perhaps hard to feed because of this. Premature babies or those who did not experience the compression of the birth canal can sometimes show quite low tone. Babywearing can again be very helpful, especially when you are physically active so that she gets a lot of tummy-to-tummy stimulation and the support of the wrap around her body. Massage can aid by stimulating organ function and the hormonal system. Again, rather than manipulate, challenge or shock your baby into a response, entice her interest. Try and meet her at her level of activity and draw her out. As she gets a bit older, resist the temptation to entertain her constantly. Instead, tantalise to awaken her desire to be active, to reach for what she wants, rather than simply lie back and wait for the fun to start. A low tone baby is so relaxed that she finds it hard to recognise that initiation from the yield in order to push away from the floor, so movement becomes difficult. If her movement skills are very delayed it would be wise to seek professional assessment through your doctor, or you could go straight to a specialist movement therapist for support if your doctor is not able to help you.

Your baby seeks safety and support. That confirmation that you are there for them is a physical act as much as an emotional feeling. Your baby needs to be able to yield her weight into your body and to feel it is welcoming and happy to connect, support and sustain her. Once that physical bond is established and your baby starts to realise that her body is actually separate from yours she will seek to bond to the earth and start to play with moving out of gravity. The rest of the year will be spent gradually working her way up and out of the floor, from belly to hands and knees and finally onto her feet. Subtle, varied and structured in a way that minimises risk, the developmental movement sequence will build her confidence by increment. Her first venture into the world outside her immediate sphere will happen with the support of the earth underneath her with the belly crawl. The only risk she faces in moving this way is what she may find on the floor as she moves forward. When she has explored the world around her for some time from this safe perspective, she will figure out how to reach and pull her body up to all fours and power forward, balancing just one knee and hand on the floor as she moves. The risk of falling enters the game, and it may take her quite a while to establish herself safely on hands and knees before she starts to move from that position. As she becomes able to travel distances she will start to sit up and watch the landscape, and search for familiar faces that she can return to when her exploring is done. And then she will reach for the environment and the space around her as support to help her move up on to her feet and complete the journey. Enjoy watching the choreography she makes.

4

PLAY DAYS
AND TOY STORY

We always learn what we experience – that which is actually happening for us. This is different from learning from our experience.

Anat Baniel, *Kids Beyond Limits*

How do you play with a baby? It's a question that I often get asked. By the time we get to adulthood, we have spent years using games, toys, words and our imaginations to play and it can be hard to envisage playing with someone who does not speak, has not yet, as far as we know, developed the ability to imagine and who has limited movement possibilities. What constitutes play with such a person? Let me give you one example of a game with a nine-week-old little client of mine.

Case study

Max is catching at my fingers, so I play the moving game. As he holds on to my fingers I gently move his arms, making funny noises as I stretch them open, out to the sides and then reach for his toes, repeating each move a few times before changing pace, energy or rhythm. He is smiling and giggling as we go. When I slow down I notice his hands want to keep going so I let him take the lead and move my whole arms where his little hands suggest they should go. We start to take turns, he leads, then me, then him again – our eyes lock in our synchronicity – we are mesmerised by his power. When he leads me I give him a big reaction, showing surprise with my voice and expression – allowing even the smallest movement to move my whole arm or even my whole body through space. He laughs and his eyes shine with excitement. When he looks over to his mother I let my own excitement subside and slowly guide his arms back down to his sides. It is time to have a rest.

Making the most of our play time with our babies can mean many different things. We can play as educators: in the example above I start in an educator role. I provide Max with specific movement experiences, then repeat, adding slight variations as I go, and give him time to notice the sensations he feels as I move his arms for him.

He is learning from this game, sensing the movement of his arms and making the connection between what he sees and what he physically feels. This will reinforce his growing awareness that he has a body all of his own. Each variation of movement gives new information to his brain; the neural network he creates in response will inform how he processes information in the future. By picking up on the initiation of movement from his hands and letting him 'move' my arms (of course I am doing the heavy lifting), I give him the satisfaction of being in charge and effecting change, supporting the idea of taking turns, demonstrating my responsiveness to his desires and reinforcing his sense of agency. In letting him take over I am telling him that I really see him, that I want to engage with him, and that he can trust me to respond to his needs and interests, I'm building a relationship with him. As I start to put more expression into my face, responding to his direction with more exaggeration and interesting sounds, I become more of an entertainer for my little friend and amuse him with surprise elements, perhaps extending the timespan of our game with this change of focus until he shows me he is tiring by looking over to his mum. I acknowledge this as our 'game over' signal and withdraw my engagement to let him rest, being present at a distance so he can call me back to play if he decides he would like to.

This is a simple playful exchange, the kind of interaction that most parents, quite appropriately, go into without any forethought – it just feels natural to play with movement, to make some sounds and funny faces, to get a reaction. I wanted to unpack that little memory for you for two reasons. Firstly so that when you find yourself playing 'making faces' or 'silly noises' or 'poking out your tongue' games with your baby, you understand that these games have value and are important. The high-pitched sing-song voice you use, the way you widen your eyes and exaggerate your facial expressions, are designed to make it easier for him to understand your communication. Clarity, pacing and repetition help him make sense of what you are doing.

You will notice that I took my cues from Max, starting with arm movements he could already make by himself, introducing the variations slowly, staying attentive and within his comfort zone so that he was successful in his efforts and was not overwhelmed. Psychologists call this skill 'attunement', and when you are attuned to your baby it is easier for you to respond appropriately to their needs and this establishes a relationship where your baby feels safe and able to thrive. Focused, physical games help you learn what amuses and interests your baby. How loud is too loud, how fast is too fast? You learn about his personality and you learn about your own levels of patience and attentiveness too. How do you prefer to play? What do you find boring and what can make it less so for you? If you are raising your child with a partner, does the way each of you plays differ? You may want to consider all that consciously and really 'think' about it, or you may be happy to simply let your subconscious do the work, relax and enjoy. It very much depends on you, how you feel, what you are used to doing, who you are. Both ways of being are equally perfect!

The second reason for my description was to illustrate some of the roles we take on when playing. Showing our babies how to do something (educator) or keeping them amused or distracted (entertainer) are often the most familiar play styles for adults. They are important aspects of play and you will use them often. I want to highlight a third style of play, however, which can be a bit more elusive when your baby is so young. It is the art of simply being a playmate. Playing with or alongside our baby is a role that is perhaps easier to imagine ourselves in when our children are older. When our toddler is able to understand or communicate with words, we can see ourselves building something or pretend baking or crafting together. But what do we do with a baby who can't speak, imagine or even move very much? Being a playmate means putting yourself in the same situation: on the same level as your child and being open to any games that evolve from that act, exploring together. In essence playing with a young baby is about connection, movement improvisation and physical experimentation. It is all about the moment, staying aware and open to sensation and the relationship between you both. We might call it the Zen of play – so how does it work?

Practically speaking, it is the act of lying down next to your baby at a distance where they can see you clearly and letting their explorations inspire your own. With a young baby it might mean simply lying next to them and watching what they watch, or making the smallest movements, just like they are. It's like taking a moment to slip inside their skin and see the world from their perspective. The simplicity of the act itself belies its significance. Mirroring your baby in its essence affirms his presence. You know you are seen when someone joins you where you are and does what you do.

One particular client was overjoyed to discover just how much her baby responded to this simple way of playing. Her son was eight weeks old and when we explored playing in this way she started by simply stretching her arm in the same way as he did. He watched her arm and seemed to understand that she was copying him. He stretched his arm again, she copied and this 'call and response' type physical game lasted for some minutes. He loved moving and then watching as his mother followed his cue. Sometimes she would lead the exchange. They played together, taking turns to watch and stretch. It was a turning point for this particular family: the following week the mother reported that her baby seemed happier and more contented since she started to spend time playing with him this way during the day and she said that she felt closer and more connected to him too.

Sometimes you will find that your baby is content in his own world while playing and you are left simply mirroring his movements, rather than interacting. Using this time for yourself is a valuable meditation, a form of mindfulness, that will build your ability to observe your baby. If you have been doing the physical explorations in this book, you will already know some of the principles you can improvise with. If your baby is stretching his arm, for example, why not explore that action at different speeds, initiating the movement from the shoulder, initiating from the fingertips. Noticing the sensations, noticing what makes the motion easier or more difficult, experimenting with pausing or flowing, with different qualities of movement. Simply being on the floor (or lying down on the bed) with your baby is a way of supporting them. In a world where everything happens in the vertical, helping your baby feel comfortable in the horizontal will encourage him to be more contented playing on his belly. The more time he spends on his belly, the more exercise his muscles get as they move in relation to gravity. If he learns to rest his head on the side, when he tires he will develop his ability to yield and push away from the floor once he is interested in moving around the space. Floor play simply makes your baby's journey up to standing smoother and less frustrating.

The other magic that floor play can perform is to give you an opportunity to rest. When you lie on your back with your baby next to you, bend your knees and put your feet on the floor near your bottom. Feel how your lower back releases towards the floor. Take a moment to simply breathe deeply and when you breathe out imagine that breath is flowing out of your body through your back surface, taking any tension out with it. Slide your shoulders down and away from your ears, or if they are particularly tense you can cross them over at the elbows above your chest to help the shoulder blades release into the floor. A few deep breaths in this position and you can refresh yourself in between your playful exchanges with your child.

If you are lying on your tummy, make sure your breasts are comfortable by placing a cushion or two just below them on your abdomen to raise your chest off the floor and avoid discomfort (especially useful if you are breastfeeding). Adults often experience stiffness in the lower back when lying on the belly, propped up on their elbows: if this is the case, focus on your lower back and try to release any tension with your breath, imagining your pelvis sinking into the floor. Make sure your arms are in a comfortable position at either side of your body and don't be afraid to simply come down to the floor and rest with your head to one side if propping yourself up on your elbows is too much of a challenge. And a quick mention for those of you who wear glasses: try to take them off when you are playing on the floor, as they get in the way of truly relaxing your head, so if you can bear not to see in the detail you are used to, try to floor play glasses free in these first few months at least.

Tummy time

Before we look at some specific ways of playing, I would like to explore the concept of 'tummy time' with you. The term itself was brought in a few years after the 'Back to Sleep' campaign, based on studies that showed a significant drop in the rate of Sudden Infant Death Syndrome (SIDS) when babies slept on their back, was adopted by health authorities all around the world. It seems that many parents decided that 'back to sleep' meant that it was dangerous for a baby to lie on their tummy at any time of day and avoided placing their babies in that position. After a few years it became apparent there had been an increase in developmental delay for babies who slept on their backs, as well as a higher incidence of flat-head syndrome.[1]

The 'tummy time' campaign was introduced to encourage parents to ensure that babies spend time playing on their tummies while they are awake. However, parents are still wary and often delay putting their babies on their tummies for several months. When they do introduce tummy time, the whole process is fraught with tension from the outset. I see parents with worried looks on their faces lifting their babies by supporting them under their armpits, and lowering their bodies, face first, towards a blanket on the floor. By the time the baby reaches the blanket they are usually crying and tense and parents soon give up on the whole idea because their baby is so distressed. If we look at this from the baby's point of view, their distress is hardly surprising. How would you feel if you suddenly found yourself 'falling' forward, face down on to the floor? As adults we have protective reflexes that mean our arms would shoot out in front of us to cushion our fall, but a baby will not develop this set of responses until they are able to crawl, so there is literally nothing they can do to save themselves – they are helpless. So, quite rightly, they get upset and the 'problem' with tummy time is born.

Some parents will just avoid tummy time for that reason. Others will feel pressure mounting from experts and friends to continue. They will suffer through several minutes every day watching a tense and unhappy baby flapping their arms and legs around while they lie on a blanket surrounded by toys they are not even remotely interested in, distressed and crying (often both parent and child!) but reassuring themselves that the baby is building strong muscles, which takes effort, and that they are doing the right thing.

There is still some discussion about the necessity of tummy time. Some baby development theories[2] suggest that a baby should not be placed in any position that they cannot achieve by themselves, arguing that there is no need for a baby to experience their tummy as a surface to lie on until they can roll on to it themselves. Others will say that babies who lie on their back all the time risk flattening the back of the skull and will take longer to develop good head control and general movement skills and it is a developmental need. While I have already argued that putting a baby in a position they are unable to reach by themselves is unhelpful, in this particular case it is not quite as black and white an issue as it may seem. While it is true that your baby cannot yet choose to lie on his tummy, he also hasn't exactly 'chosen' to lie on his back. Parents make those initial choices and there are good developmental reasons to ensure that your baby experiences the world through all the surfaces of his body, not just his back. From a somatic perspective it is important that a baby has an experience of lying on all the surfaces of his body, not just to encourage muscles to strengthen, but also in order to support movement development in a more subtle way.

In the last chapter we spoke about the tissue tone of a baby, and how extremes of high and low general tone can make it more difficult for a baby to progress through movement because it requires more energy to move from a place of tension or collapse and it can feel very uncomfortable. One of the ways that the tone of our baby's body is developed is in relation to gravity. When we lie on our belly or back, the surface in contact with the floor responds to gravity by moving towards it. So when we are on our belly the flexor tone of our body is activated as the muscles on the front of our body are drawn down by gravity, helping the belly release and relax into the floor, and supporting the ability to yield and eventually push up with the torso on the in breath, away from the floor. When lying on the back the extensor tone is supported and the muscles of our back create an opposite arc of tension.

If we spend all our time on our back, the extensor tone becomes stronger than the flexor tone and an imbalance is created, which will underlie further movement development. This will make it harder for your baby to crawl and sit up independently. Lying on the side of our bodies needs support from flexors and extensors to sustain the balance, as different areas are drawn by gravity, allowing some structures to release, others to strengthen. When babies regularly experience lying on front, back and sides it will help to establish a balanced tone throughout their bodies, so that the connective tissue, muscles and bones that move us learn to cooperate easily, efficiently and offer your baby a full range of motion to choose from.

But then here you are with a totally curled up bundle of a newborn whose tummy wouldn't even touch the floor if you put them there. The internet is talking tummy time, but to be perfectly honest there doesn't seem to be much point in placing them on the floor and I agree. If we model what our baby needs to learn on the pattern that underlies our movement – that yield, push, reach and pull – it seems that we need to establish the possibility of a yield into gravity before we have a hope of pushing up and away from it. So the point of giving your newborn time on their tummy is not to encourage them to tense and lift their head (although they will do so reflexively at first), it is, in the first instance, all about them finding a way to *rest* in that position, their head turned to the side. This act alone will help prepare them to move their head and neck with control.

Taking into consideration your baby's physical need to be close to you, it makes total sense to introduce tummy time to your baby by rolling them out of your arms on to your belly while you lie down. It is as simple as that: skin-to-skin (baby in a nappy, you bare chested), relaxing together. You may need to gently turn your baby's head to one side so he can comfortably rest it on one cheek, but make sure that you alternate the direction he is looking in.

If you are breastfeeding it can be a bit uncomfortable, as breasts are still getting used to their milk production in the first few weeks and just the smell of the milk can make a baby restless sometimes. So this particular tummy time activity can be easier for Dads or other family members to try out and it is a nice way to bond, especially if there is chest hair involved for your baby to explore! Just resting one hand on your baby's bottom as he lies on your chest will anchor him securely and help him yield his weight. The key to helping your baby feel happy in this position is to feel relaxed and comfortable yourself (enough pillows!), and to either engage his attention by smiling, cooing or whispering sweet nothings, or if he is sleepy just letting him rest while you take some time to relax.

Once this becomes a familiar position for you to play and relax in, you might roll on to your side with your baby so that you are both lying on your sides to play and then you can help him roll on to his tummy from his side. If you lie down with your face beside him or opposite, at the same level, and sing or speak or play, this should reassure him. It is an activity to enjoy together little and often, just until he starts to squirm or seems to have had enough. Whether that is two minutes or ten is fine, just repeat it regularly throughout the day. Don't think of it as endurance training! When he gets tense and uncomfortable you have lost the yield and there is no need to continue, so gently roll him back to his side, pause for a minute or so to give him time to register and respond and either stay there or continue on to his back or into your arms. If your baby continues to seem unhappy on his belly, make sure you have checked out practical considerations. Perhaps the surface is too soft and he feels he is sinking and stuck. Does he know that he can put his head down on one side to rest, and that it is not just about holding your head up and looking? Is the umbilical cord tie uncomfortable or pressing into his belly?

Comfort is key here – yours and your baby's. If you are not comfortable, or are worried in any way, then your baby will read that signal loud and clear. If it is hard for you to lie on the floor with your baby then at this newborn stage you can place them on a higher surface: bed, changing table or the dinner table and sit on a chair to bring you face-to-face with them. Pay attention to how you put your baby on to their tummy. Slowly rolling from the back to their side, waiting until they are settled and only then continuing on to the belly will create a smoother, more gradual transition for them. Make sure you never leave your baby unsupervised in this position of course, even for a moment.

Usually your baby will prefer to watch your face, but if you show him toys, be aware of the level at which you hold them. If you hold them high then your baby has to strain their neck to see and they may not be ready to do so. A great floor play game to enjoy together is 'spider fingers'. Just scuttle your fingers from side to side, or towards him or away, on the surface of the floor or table, encouraging him to turn his head in both directions. Any ordinary household object will interest your baby: sounds, songs and words will work just as well.

Some babies totally love being on their belly; it can be really soothing if they have wind or digestive issues. Some prefer the floor/bed to their parents' bodies and vice versa. Some babies never really seem to enjoy it until they can roll. If your baby is getting distressed he will become tense and unable to yield to gravity, which defeats the whole object and causes stress, so try some alternatives instead. These babies can benefit a lot from babywearing, as this will stimulate the front of their body surface through contact with you. They may also enjoy lying over your knees/thighs on their tummy, or if you carry them with their belly resting on your forearm. It is a good idea to continue offering tummy time every day or two, but setting up a stressful association is unhelpful so stay relaxed, don't leave him in distress and respect your baby's limits.

Games to play with your newborn

One of the pleasures of parenting is coming up with games to play with your baby. That moment when your baby's eyes sparkle with joy or understanding that the fun has begun is very precious. It's a personal and creative process, instinctive and joyful. However, when you are having a hard day or the sleep deprivation kicks in it can be hard to get creative. It's not all on you and instead of feeling a responsibility to initiate every game and interaction, there is value in allowing your baby to instigate the interaction, and to set the pace of their arousal. Play is an intensive activity for your baby, and it will not and should not take up all his waking hours. Short bursts of intimate play will be balanced by long hours of holding, feeding and carrying without particularly intensive face-to-face time. Ideally there will be some periods of time every day when your baby is lying with you on the floor on tummy, back and sides with space and freedom to move his arms and legs as he wishes. As your baby matures he may also be happy and content lying down and listening and watching you and the world as it goes about its business. Here are a few games that support various aspects of development and relationships that you can try out, add to and adapt as you will. Have fun!

Follow the impulse

Go gently – this is one to try from around eight weeks of age.
If you hold your baby out in front of you with one hand behind his head and the other holding his bottom you can amplify his spinal movements and let them carry him through space. Make sure you are watching and interacting with him joyfully and when he starts to wriggle let the impulse feed through your hands and move him in space in the direction he is trying to go in. It can be a very satisfying feeling for him to sense his impulse to move take him further than he could manage by himself. A baby normally has little choice in when, where or how he is moved and placed, so the feeling of actually directing where you want to go can be very pleasurable and offer him new movement ideas he may explore later on when alone.

Body sounds

With baby on his back, hold his hands or feet and gently move them, making funny noises to go with each move:

touch his nose with a 'peep', make a rumbling sound as you circle the arms... whatever takes your fancy. Watch him smile! As your baby reaches 8–12 weeks of age focus on movements that acquaint his hands and feet with each other to support his ability to come into the midline, organising his body in relation to the central axis of his spine.

Turn-taking game

By the end of three months your baby will be combining navel radiation with spinal movements and be increasingly interested in your relationship, so in addition to all the cooing and smiling and tongue-poking out games that ensue, try the turn-taking game that I described at the start of this chapter.

When your baby is lying on his back and moving his limbs and you are facing him, gently press your thumbs into the palm of his hands. This will make him reflexively grasp your thumbs and you can gently and slowly move his arms apart and together. Do not force the movement, just take it as far as is easy. Once he has got the idea, you can explore other movements of the arms – circles, spirals, whatever you like. Go slow, go gentle, repeat the same movement a few times before changing or pausing. Never force his arms if he is resisting a movement. Watch his face carefully and be sensitive to the possibility that he might initiate some movements by himself. When you feel the slightest impulse from him, allow it to move your arms, or even your whole body... giving him a massive response or conclusion to his movement impulse. As he starts to get to know the game, be generous in your turn-taking, and amplify the effect of his tiny initiations with your body and your face. He will love having a big impact on the world around him, seeing his intention taken all the way through to a big result. You in turn will train your awareness and responsiveness to his signals in a playful way.

Toys for the first three months

Tempting as it is to fill your baby's world with all the cute and interesting toys that are around, in the first three months you will get little reward for your purchases. For the first four to eight weeks at least, your baby simply needs to find out that he has a body and that it is separate to everything around him, and get used to this new environment he has joined. He will gaze at anything that catches his attention; for example sharp contrasts of tone, such as a shadow on a wall or if you have dark hair. You might be intrigued to find him gazing at your hairline instead of your eyes. Toys are pretty much irrelevant to your baby's primary task, which is simply to get used to being here and working out that he has a body and what it feels like.

Once your baby has established his own physical presence, at some stage during the second to the fourth month, his main attention will be on his relationship to you. Psychologists call this phase 'core relatedness'. Your baby will start to differentiate between objects and his parents. He will gaze intently at your face, noticing every micro expression and every response you make. He will try to copy your expressions and start to make the active mouth movements and vocalisations that we call 'pre-speech'. At some point you will get a real 'eyes-locked' smile. For many parents this is when they start to see their baby's personality more clearly. You may find that when you try to interest him in a toy he will spend the time watching your face rather than watching the toy itself. As with everything about development, this is a phase and this period will also fade from the foreground as he starts to discover objects and crawling. Face-to-face games will make the most of this special time, and anything that repeats will enthrall him. Walking our fingers through the air to 'beep' his nose, or bending down with a whooshing sound to kiss his chin can endlessly amuse.

Towards the end of our three-month time frame your baby will go from simply looking at a toy to holding it and probably sucking it, so although any household object can function as a toy, choose your items carefully. Some of the early 'toys' I use in sessions are natural bristle brushes (new of course), hair curlers of all types, pine cones and empty plastic pots and bottles (you can put a bit of rice or coloured water in a bottle to create more interest).

In the early weeks your baby's hearing is more developed than his eyesight, so making sounds, singing and speaking to your baby may well be more interesting to him than looking at things. As his eyes and hands start to become more active, at around eight to twelve weeks, toys and objects with interesting textures to feel become useful. Find a variety of textures for him to lie on: blankets, play mats, rugs and towels will all do the trick. And by the end of three months objects that are light and a bit more intricate become popular. Your baby will most likely be reaching for and holding toys above his body, exploring what he needs to do to reach the part of the toy that he is interested in. Interlocking wooden rings of various colours are a great favourite and can be played with on the tummy or when lying on the back.

My favourite way of choosing something that a baby can play with is to simply spend a minute or two exploring the item myself. Feel the texture, the weight, does it make any noise as you move it, how does it feel on the skin of your cheek? Play with it with your eyes shut for a while as well as open, what do you notice? Getting used to offering your baby the chance to join in with some of your everyday activities is also a nice way to build your relationship and offer learning opportunities. Offer your baby the same object you are using, a post-it note, the carrot peel, a sock, a blade of grass... show your baby the world and share his wonder!

A word about screens. Guidelines issued by the American Academy of Pediatrics advise that children under the age of 18 months should not spend any time at all watching screens.[3] Apart from taking time away from opportunities for learning through play and relationships, their eyes are still developing two important abilities: depth of vision and the ability to track a moving object. This happens as they watch the world around them and their eyes alternate focus from near to far. Watching a flat two-dimensional screen image is detrimental to this process. This has implications for you and your screen use. Your baby wants to learn how to be an adult and if smartphone and laptop use is a major part of the adult activity they see, that is what they will want to be doing as soon as they can make their preferences clear. Minimising your own screen use when your baby is awake and attentive is worth consideration, even at this early stage.

5

NAILING THE
DAY-TO-DAY

'I felt like I was being hit over the head with a baseball bat and winning the lottery at the same time…'
Koni, Expatbabies Berlin

Now you understand the principles of development as a base to work from, and you can better assess what your baby needs to experience generally, let's get down to the more mundane and everyday. This chapter is about the nitty-gritty of daily life: feeding, sleeping, managing your expectations, making and revising decisions at a time when you are potentially full of anxiety and sleep deprived – the 'just keeping it all going' bit. What will my life be like once the baby is here? It's the big unknown that it is hard to prepare for before the birth: how will you feel physically and mentally? What will your baby be feeling? We can't answer those questions, but we can look at the kinds of issues you may find yourself dealing with so that if they come up for you they don't come as a total surprise. There are negatives and positives in every situation. The quotations you will see in this chapter are the real-life responses I received when I asked mums in the Expatbabies Berlin Facebook group to describe what parenting a newborn baby was like for them. Real and honest and so very varied, they illustrate how individual the experience is for each of us. I hope that this chapter gives you a realistic idea of the issues, decisions and experiences that many new parents find themselves dealing with in the first three months of family life, as well as some useful tips and resources to help you navigate your way through with at least a sense of ease and good humour.

Expectations

'Have you established a routine yet?' I think this is the number one question that is guaranteed to make a mother feel small, guilty or a complete failure. Routine is talked about like it is some kind of holy grail of parenting... once you have established a routine, all will be well, the implication being that if you can't achieve a routine you have somehow failed at parenting. This annoys me, big time. It simply doesn't take account of the way needs vary and it can make parents who are responsive to the changing needs of their baby feel like failures when they are, in fact, doing a wonderful job.

I think this concept has its roots back in the 1950s, the high point of patriarchal interest in maternity, when bottle-feeding was the best you could do for your baby and 'scientifically' set timetables for feeding, napping and exercise were quoted like mantras. That was a long time ago. And whether hearing 'routine' thrills you with its promise of order and certainty, or makes you feel constrained and bored, we need to see its value through the lens of what we now know. The basic principle of attachment, being responsive to our child's needs and meeting them as often as possible, is paramount in establishing our child's psychological wellbeing. Just think about how much changes for your baby in this first year, how fast their brain and body are growing in skill and understanding, how new everything is and how easily their senses can be overwhelmed. How on earth is keeping to a strict timetable without regard to those changes going to be responsive?

To be fair, most people would not expect a newborn to be in a routine, especially if being breastfed, as feeding on demand means just that: feeding your child whenever they indicate that they are hungry. However, by three months you might start to experience internal or external pressure to create a clear structure for the day. Too often this implies that you should try to change your child's natural behaviour, and get them to nap and sleep at set times or for a set number of hours per day. While it may work out for a few weeks, you will inevitably feel a failure at some point if you think that the matter is settled for good. Your baby's physical growth does not happen like the gently curved line on a graph… there are growth spurts, during which she will feed non-stop. The chance of illness, teething (yes, some babies get their first teeth very early) and all sorts of potential disruptions will ensure that any timetable you set cannot be fulfilled. Why not let yourself off that particular hook? Instead of putting your energy into managing your child's behaviour because the books say it should be done one particular way, focus instead on getting to know your particular baby and how they show you what they need. Let's redraw this concept of parenting routine and think of it as a process of finding your rhythm together. A rhythm can be very regular, and that may suit you both really well, but it is not set in stone. It is co-created and responsive, able to change fluidly to meet the inevitable changes ahead.

It is easy to get caught up in a research frenzy about optimum feeding and sleeping arrangements. The sense of responsibility for another's life can hit some of us pretty hard, and that is perfectly normal. I want to help you keep things in perspective. The optimum situation is that your baby gets enough sleep and nutrition to thrive physically and emotionally. Furthermore, optimum is not just about your baby: optimum means that you, the parents, also have enough sleep, food and company to keep body and soul together. If you are feeling well supported you will be more able to cope with the demands of parenting. If you are coping, your baby copes better too. It is that simple.

All the details, which have the tendency to consume

our thoughts and discussions, will be different for every family. Will you use a moses basket, cot or co-sleep? Is it better to breast or bottle-feed? Nappies: disposable, washable or no nappy at all? There is no 'right' answer. Some of the decisions you make will be in line with 'best practice' and will get you professional or community approval, some won't. Some will suit your baby perfectly and work out, some decisions you will have to revise. Getting the most benefit for your baby, whatever choices you make, is my priority in this chapter. It is your family, they are your decisions, and the sooner you get used to making and possibly revising your own parenting decisions the better.

However used to decision-making you may be, it can be difficult when it comes to your baby. Here is a visualisation to help you at times when you might feel overwhelmed. It will calm you and help you tune into the wisdom of your body to support you in your thinking. Use it when contradictory information or strong opinions come at you from all directions and it's just too much, or when you start doubting your choices and feeling judged by others. Clear thinking is hard when you are feeling emotionally overwhelmed or upset, so instead of ignoring your emotions and trying to battle through with logic, take a few minutes to address them from a different perspective. Whether you make your decision based on the research evidence or your gut feeling, or a combination of the two, it is important to acknowledge the emotions the decision brings up in you and feel comfortable with your choice.

Exercise: Settling your brain

Lie down on your back with your knees bent and feet on the floor. Allow your eyelids to close. Welcome the support of the earth.

Imagine all the thoughts and feelings that are worrying you buzzing around within you – use a physical image. They could be snowflakes swirling, autumn leaves in the wind, a sandstorm, surf crashing onto rocks, post-it notes... find an image that you can connect with easily. I will use the word 'thoughts'.

Visualise the thoughts start to slow down and settle, inside you, drawn by gravity.

Watch them settle within the soles of your feet. Feel them sinking into the bowl of your pelvis, filling it up half way.

All along your back, the round bones of your vertebrae are just showing through the surface, like the peaks of some forgotten mountain range.

Feel your thoughts settle inside the lower portion of your neck.

Sense the globe that is your skull, and imagine the thoughts settling at the base, filling it up to the ears.

Take a moment to scan and enjoy this beautiful, still landscape.

Notice your breath, how it flows through your body. Imagine that the air comes in through your navel and flows simultaneously up and down your spine, returning to the navel to leave on your out breath.

Take a few breaths feeling this movement – breathe the air in and fill your spine, then let it flow back out and away from the navel once again.

Enjoy locating this midline of your body with your breath.

Feel the calm stillness inside your body.

Now let's focus on your decision. With your elbow resting comfortably on the floor, place one hand on your gut. Breathe into your gut and say hello to it inside your mind. Ask it how it feels about the issue. Note the feelings, images or sensations you perceive.

Now place the other hand on your heart. Connect to your heart, say hello. Ask it how it feels about the issue. Note the feelings, images or sensations.

Leaving your hands in connection with gut and heart, focus on the brain and imagine the breath flowing up the centre of your body, linking gut, heart and brain.

Say hello to your brain, thank it for working so hard and remind it there are other structures in the body, like the heart and the gut, that are there to support it.

Ask your brain how it feels about the issue. Note the response, feelings, images or sensations.

Imagine the breath flowing up the centre of your body, connecting gut, heart and brain, sharing.

When you are ready, focus your attention on the clear spaces within your body, the air above your settled thoughts.

Feel the lightness in the upper parts of your body. Sense the space in your toes, your legs, your knees. Feel the space at the front of your belly, your sternum, ribs and the surface of your heart. Imagine the space in the front of your shoulders, your upper chest and neck. Sense the space within your face, your jaw, your nose, your eyes, your forehead.

As you connect to the space and light inside your body, let your body move in response and allow your eyes to open to the world. Get up slowly to sitting.

As you come up to sitting, notice how your body feels now. Notice how your brain feels. Did you get some clear messages from your gut and your heart, or was one or the other hard to connect to? It may surprise you that we nave neural tissue in some of our organs, not just in our brains and nervous system, so connecting the gut, heart and brain is not as 'away with the fairies' as you may have first thought. You may have had a very strong perception from one or other of the areas you focused on, or it may simply be that your brain is better able to relax as it feels the support of the other organs. The more you use this visualisation, the easier it will be to feel that visceral support for your cortical processes.

The only time I found it hard was when I listened to other people rather than my baby.

Andrea, Expatbabies Berlin

Let's take a look at the two major decisions that every parent is faced with: how you feed your baby and what the sleeping arrangements will be.

Feeding

The choice between breast or bottle-feeding your baby is often not a choice at all. While we know that breastmilk is the healthiest option for baby and mother, it can sometimes be hard to establish a happy breastfeeding relationship. It is also a valid choice to bottle-feed your baby for medical reasons or simply because that is what you prefer. This book is not about judging people's choices. Let's focus instead on making the many hours of your day that you spend feeding your baby as comfortable and relaxing and as beneficial to your baby's development as possible.

Before we get practical I would like to explain why, at

least for the first few weeks, it is not possible to simply alternate feeding methods as you wish and then make a decision. Part of it is you, and part your baby. Your body relies on the information it gets from your baby to regulate itself to her needs – breastmilk composition and quantity is tailored to your specific baby, so the best way to ensure that your body produces the appropriate amount of milk is to ensure that breastmilk is your baby's only food source. From your baby's perspective, alternating feeding methods (in particular alternating breast and bottle-feeding before the breastfeeding is well established) can make it difficult for them to breastfeed due to nipple confusion. It all comes down to the action of suckling/sucking, because breasts and nipples are not at all like teats and bottles, however similar they may look.

Suckling a nipple is a whole body action in which the baby reaches and opens the mouth utilising the top portion of the jaw as well as the bottom. It is a big movement that requires energy. The head rocks back and forth slightly as a baby suckles and this massage moves sequentially down the spine. The suckle itself is initiated by a reach of the upper part of the jaw and your nipple finds itself vacuum packed against your baby's soft palate, while their lips and gums stimulate the breast tissue and milk ducts to flow, regulating it by pumping at first and then resting while the milk flows into the mouth.

Sucking the teat of a bottle is a much smaller action, and the movement happens mainly in the lower jaw. The flow is relatively regular, and when a baby sucks they taste milk, and when they stop, it stops. If you introduce a bottle before breastfeeding is established, you may find your baby finds the bottle easier and prefers it to the breast. Similarly, if you wait too long, the bottle may be rejected because of its unfamiliarity (even if it is full of your expressed breastmilk). So it can be a little tricky finding the perfect moment to introduce a bottle, if that's what you decide to do. Some breastfed babies will happily accept a bottle of expressed milk on occasion, but some are very reluctant and some parents give up trying because it is too difficult. Once again all families are different! Don't despair if your carefully laid plans need to be revised, and remember that you can seek help from your health visitor, infant feeding team or breastfeeding support organisations (they will happily discuss introducing a bottle with you, and will not judge you!)

If your wish is to breastfeed and you encounter problems at the start, making it necessary for your baby to experience alternative feeding, it may be advisable to use a supplementary nursing system (SNS), which consists of a bottle attached to a thin tube that is taped next to your nipple, so your baby suckles as in breastfeeding, but gets milk from the bottle. It is also possible for a newborn baby to be fed with a cup, taking small sips of expressed milk or formula if needed, so that it is easier for them to accept the breast later on. If you are bottle-feeding, have a look at 'paced bottle-feeding' as a way of ensuring that you are feeding your baby as responsively as possible.

Whether you are breast or bottle-feeding, here are

some ways that you can optimise the benefits your baby receives from this time you spend together.

Development-friendly feeding tips

- Use the rooting reflex as a way to find out if your baby is truly hungry and to set up a good latch if breastfeeding. If your baby is hungry and you stroke the area around their lips in one direction, they will turn their face in that direction if they are hungry, and open their mouth wide in expectation of finding milk. It promotes a good latch if you are breastfeeding, and whichever way you feed if your baby does not respond to stimulation around their mouth it is unlikely that they are hungry (the label 'reflex' is a bit misleading). If you have managed to anticipate their hunger and your baby is relatively calm, then it is a great way to start your feed. With your baby in your arm on her back, stroke your nipple or the teat of the bottle from the corner of her lips out to her cheek (on the side that is nearest your body). Your baby will turn her head to find the milk and you can turn her body as soon as she has latched on so that she is in the tummy-to-tummy position for her actual feed.

- Make sure you alternate the side of your body that you feed your baby on. Your baby needs to experience this regular position on both sides of her body. This is especially important to note for bottle-feeding parents, as you will likely find one side of your body more comfortable than the other and might tend to always feed on that side. Use a sticker on your clothes or a bracelet that you switch to the side which you need to feed on next time after each feed. When breastfeeding either you will be emptying both breasts during a feed, or alternating one side then the other because one will be fuller than the other, so it's a bit easier to remember to do this.

- To help stimulate a stronger suckle (which can be useful if your baby is premature or particularly sleepy and gets tired easily when feeding):

  » make sure her knees are bent/legs flexed and her bottom is lower than her head.

  » massage the soles of her feet with a rhythmic pressing-pumping action, or simply ensure they are pressed into your elbow/the side of the chair/sofa so that she feels a pressure on her feet and she will pump herself.

  » relax – yes, I mean you! Relax, breathe deep, lean back or lie down, and make sure your arm is supported by cushions so you can transmit this relaxation to your baby. This in turn will help her feed more calmly and digest her food better, a win-win.

  » make sure that your baby's head is supported on the side so you are not restricting her ability to rock her head backwards if she is breastfeeding.

- Use feeding as a time to connect with your little one. She is at the distance where she can see you most clearly, so give her your attention when she wants it.

You might find your baby is sleepy after a feed or that it is her awake and alert time, so meet her mood and enjoy her.

- Help your baby to produce gas or a burp after they have fed by holding them vertically with their belly supported against your body, support their head with one hand and with the other massage their lower back in circles, up and down or in a small jiggling action side to side. Other methods include holding them tightly against your body in this position and making big movements up and down or side to side yourself, to help any air bubbles work their way out. I never found patting on the back very useful, but some people recommend it so it's something you might try.

Making breastfeeding work for you

Breastfeeding is how we are designed to feed our children, so it should be easy, right? For many people it is a wonderful and happy experience from the start. For others it can be more of a struggle. Successful breastfeeding is very dependent on your expectations, the quality of your birth experience and on the support you have to enable you to both get started and continue with it. If your birth is uncomplicated and your baby is simply wiped dry after birth and placed skin-to-skin on your belly, she will initiate breastfeeding all by herself. It can be a slow process, with your baby taking little rests along the way as she wiggles up your belly to find your breast, like a little caterpillar. If you support your baby's feet and make sure you are lying horizontally, it will make it easier. When she reaches your breast your baby will use her hands and mouth to find your nipple and latch on for her first feed. This process is beautifully shown in action in the film *The Moving Child*.[1] This reflexive crawl and feed can almost be seen as a completion of the birth process for your baby – your baby, in the world, taking what she needs and wants for herself.

In terms of your body, your breasts will also take some time to acclimatise to their new role. The first type of breastmilk they produce, known as colostrum, is a superfood high in protein, fat-soluble vitamins, minerals and immunoglobulins, to ensure that even if your baby is struggling to learn to feed what they do manage to ingest is extra-nutritious. You may hear colostrum referred to as 'liquid gold' or 'the first vaccination', as it helps to kick-start the baby's immune system. If you plan to bottle-feed, you might consider giving your baby the colostrum, either by feeding at the breast or by expressing and feeding it via syringe, to ensure your baby has this first dose of immune-boosting milk. After about three to four days the composition of your milk changes, your breasts will feel harder and may be uncomfortable and warm for a day or two until a feeding pattern is established and they work out how much milk to produce for your baby. Many mothers worry about whether their breasts are producing enough milk, even when their babies are putting on weight steadily (after the initial post-birth weight loss, which happens to all babies in the first few days). Once breastfeeding is established you will find that your breasts will feel fuller as it becomes time to feed your child, and they may even leak when you see her or pick her up for a feed. That is how in tune your body is with your baby!

If you have a breastfeeding support group in your area it is a good idea to visit while you are still pregnant. Just seeing how other people feed and hearing their experiences is helpful and will make you feel more comfortable when it's your turn. Meeting the person who is leading the group can give you a head start if you experience any difficulties. They will be a familiar person to turn to for advice. If you do experience difficulties and your midwife or health visitor cannot help (they have some training, but may be very stretched for time) then it is a very good idea to contact a breastfeeding counsellor or lactation consultant and have a consultation as soon as possible. This is not something to delay: you feed your baby so many times a day that dreading the process will make it difficult for you and your baby to establish a secure bond. There are some useful resources listed at the back of this book.

Another thing to remember – and this is important information for those people around you – is that breastfeeding is a *job*. You need extra rest and good nutrition to support your recovery and enable you to feed your baby round the clock. You need to be supported in this by those who are close to you and this can be part of their role in the early days. Try to ensure that you have access to healthy, nutritious snacks and drinks to keep you going throughout the day and night. Apart from making you extra hungry, breastfeeding makes you sleepy, as the hormones it releases are feel-good, relaxed hormones. Especially in the early weeks it is a good idea to establish a feeding corner in your home, equipped with everything you may need to have to hand while you feed... food, drink, tissues, something to listen to if you are feeling a bit lonely, lots of cushions to prop your head and elbows. As you get more used to feeding it becomes easier and easier, but for now the comfort of simply having everything you need to keep yourself and your baby happy cannot be underestimated!

Not all first time babies are challenging... You can get lucky! My baby slept for 16 hours per day, ate really well and was a dream in the first three months! Stephanie

Sleep baby, sleep!

While we may hear tales of babies that sleep in eight-hour stretches, the chances are that your baby will not. Newborn care is a 24-hour activity and, at the very start at least, there is not much difference between night and day for your baby. Some babies do sleep for longer stretches than others, or simply wake, feed and sleep without fuss, but others find it hard to settle back to sleep after feeding, or have difficulty sleeping at all. No one can tell you what your baby will be like and it will usually take some time to find some kind of sustainable sleep solution for you all.

The one clear rhythm you need to set from the start

is that there is a difference between night and day. This means marking evening with a change in atmosphere and less stimulation. This can be tricky if you have a partner who only gets to see their baby after work, and ramps up the excitement just before 'bedtime'. Take this into consideration when you start to set that evening mood. You would be surprised at the number of parents who guiltily admit to me that their baby goes to bed when they do and much later than their particular cultural 'norm'. It's one of those decisions that depends on what your lifestyle demands, as well as what your baby needs. Getting some sleep is the important factor here, for both you and your baby. Where and when you do it is much less important than getting enough of it!

Whenever you decide night time starts, feeding your baby during this time should involve the lowest level of light you can manage with, the least disturbance possible and minimal talking. If your baby is wide awake and wanting to play, be less responsive than you would be in the daytime. It will not damage her development to find that there is a difference between the night and day reactions from her parents. I write this in the full knowledge that you will undoubtedly give in to the little smiley, cooing individual from time to time, who can resist...? But give it a few weeks of broken sleep and it becomes easier. As your baby matures into the fourth month and accepts the night and day rhythm and her tummy can take in larger amounts of milk, you will want her to feed less frequently at night than during the daytime. To support that make sure that her daytimes offer her plenty of opportunities to feed calmly, without distraction, in between a nice range of play, movement and social experiences.

Sensible sleeping for night-feeding parents

If you are responsible for waking up to feed your baby at night, it is highly unlikely that you will get your full quota of sleep at night time. Most of us manage fine for a few days or weeks with reduced sleep, but this is a long-term occupation and you need to find ways to recharge your energy. If you are breastfeeding, you will be solely in charge of night-time feeds for at least the first few weeks, although once breastfeeding is well established using expressed milk in a bottle may be a good way to share the load with a partner. Napping or at least consciously resting during the day is therefore a really important skill to foster.

If napping is difficult you need to work out why. In the first few days it is not unusual for sleeping to be an issue: you may be high with excitement or worry... you worry if your baby is noisy when they sleep and if they are silent, you find yourself watching them intently to make sure they are still breathing. If that is making it difficult to sleep then you need some help, and this is where partners, family and friends can step in. Alternatively you might pay for a babysitter to simply sit with your baby in another room while you rest, safe in the knowledge that the baby is being cared for by someone else. This may not be as easy as it sounds, and it can be hard to relinquish responsibility for someone so precious to you, but it is well worth making the effort. Rest will make you a better parent; you resting is a way to care for your child.

However tired you are, a nap might be difficult to achieve. If you find it hard to sleep in the daytime, don't set your sights too high. Start by trying to simply rest while your baby sleeps (or your partner/babysitter takes her for a walk). You might simply lie down in your bedroom, curtains drawn so it is properly dark, and listen to music for a while simply trying to clear your mind. The 'Being Inside' visualisation on page 32 offers a way to get into a more relaxed state of mind, or perhaps you have a favourite relaxation or meditation recording to listen to. The more regularly you rest, the easier it will be to sleep. Pay attention to the number of caffeinated drinks or sugary snacks you eat, and try to avoid them for a few hours before you have your rest. If your baby is one who needs to be held almost all the time, it can be really challenging to use the time you have without them in your arms to rest. I remember very clearly the confusion that would set in when my firstborn finally dropped off and let herself be put down in the moses basket. Did I pee, eat or sleep first? It was a difficult choice to make for me at the time!

If you are bottle-feeding your baby you need your rest too, but hopefully you also have more options in terms of sharing responsibility for feeding her with others. The key task you have is to actually make sure it happens! That may not be as easy as it seems. Some new mums will find it hard to leave their baby in someone else's care, even if that person is the baby's other parent, while some will be feeling lonely for adult company and need that more than they feel they need their sleep. Partners may have responsibilities that make waking at night impractical to arrange. Remember that these broken nights will go on for a long time, so it really is worth finding an arrangement that will enable you to get more than two hours sleep at a stretch for a few days per week. Setting it up right from the start is much easier than waiting until you are exhausted and desperate. Some things you can consider are temporarily sleeping separately from your partner, having them get up early with the baby when they are not working, or staying up late with the baby while you go to bed for a couple of hours earlier in the evening.

This is the hardest thing I have done in my life. I have never felt so uninformed, afraid, tired, unprepared... but when I look back I feel I have become stronger and that whatever works is good for you and your baby. Don't hesitate to ask for help. Cristina

Where should my baby sleep?

Welcome to one of those contentious baby topics. You will either have a very clear idea of the type of sleeping arrangements you want, or you are going to spend much of your time researching. Most articles you see will agree on two things: one, that the best position for your baby to sleep in is on their back, and two, that the best place for a baby to sleep until around six months of age is in the same room as their parents. That is about all the agreement you are going to get, and even that is open to debate. See the further reading section at the back of the book for more. You will find researchers arguing that co-sleeping puts your baby in danger, and others telling you it is actually safer to have your baby sleeping with you. You will meet people who will happily let their babies sleep on their bellies, and those who will never place their baby on their tummy at any time day or night. Some babies find it very difficult to sleep on their back and whatever the parents' initial intentions they end up sleeping on their belly, or in their bed, or in a separate cot because they find it less disturbing. If you are co-parenting and your opinions differ it can be very difficult, especially if your baby finds it difficult to sleep in the situation you end up agreeing on.

Unfortunately, following national guidelines gives no guarantees, although it minimises the chance of something bad happening. Fortunately, the risk of SIDS is very, very small. In 2015 the Office of National Statistics recorded a rate of 0.27 deaths per 1,000 live births in England and Wales. The causes of SIDS are unknown, and while we call it a 'syndrome' that doesn't mean there is one cause for all cases. The most likely explanation is that there are multiple factors that when they occur together might be devastating. You can only do your best with the information you have. Given this sobering fact, it is important that your decisions are informed and considered – if you have done your research and still have questions, ask your health providers for evidence-based information to support their advice. At the end of the day, making a decision that is considered and informed, so that you can live with its consequences, is the only way you can go: no one can predict the future. Make your peace with the situation you all decide upon, because there will be many more such decisions waiting on your parenting journey.

Giving birth and having a newborn reconnects us to the very roots of our species and as mothers we learn to finally trust our instincts, which are incredibly powerful.
Halina, Expatbabies Berlin

Living the day-to-day

Cuddle, play, feed, change, sleep, repeat. That's it – the five activities that will make up your days with your baby for the next few months. At some point within the first few weeks you will add a walk in the fresh air to the list. So the pattern of your day will be some kind of order of feed, sleep, change, cuddle, play and walk and repeat. For weeks on end. You may be in a position to do this full-time, or you might find yourself returning to paid work within weeks of giving birth. Whatever the situation, the demands on you: your energy, your emotions, your patience and your physical wellbeing are substantial, especially in the first few months. While many new mums feel external pressure or an internal need to get back to 'normal' as fast as possible, acknowledging this time of transition is important. Yes, women can do anything, but when we try to do everything at the same time, we run the risk of burnout.

The idea of setting aside a specific amount of time after the birth in which new mothers are offered intensive support from their community and their loved ones is one that has existed for centuries. In many cultures around the world it is still practised. In Germany it's called the Wochenbett, in the UK the babymoon or historically a 'lying in' period. When you consider that your baby needs to acclimatise to the world gradually to avoid overwhelm, it makes sense to shield them a bit from the big wide world and stagger their introduction somewhat. In Germany midwives often suggest that mothers plan to spend a week *in* the bed, a week *on* the bed, a week in their apartment and a week venturing out occasionally into their local neighbourhood. In the UK it is normal for your midwife to visit you at home for around 10 days to check on your recovery and that of your baby, rather than expecting you to travel. It's not just your baby who will benefit from a few weeks of rest. There are good physical and psychological reasons to take it easy and allow yourself to be 'looked after' after birth, although if you are riding high on a wave of euphoria with your new baby in your arms you may find it hard to accept.

> *I honestly thought my baby would sleep all day and I'd have time to go the museum, read a book, work out – ha ha. I've only managed to read two books since Oscar was born... and he's almost two!* Juliana, Expatbabies Berlin

Making the most of your babymoon

Rest is so undervalued in today's society and is about to become very precious to you. Your body has worked hard and rest is needed for it to heal and recover. The placenta which your baby made to sustain itself leaves a wound about 22cm in diameter on the wall of your uterus, which takes around 4–6 weeks to heal. The tissue of your vagina and perineal area has stretched, possibly grazed and torn, and it may feel bruised and sore for some time. The lining of your uterus is leaving your body, like a heavy period. You may have spent several weeks with sleep interrupted, your labour may have felt long and arduous, and that is just an uncomplicated vaginal birth. A c-section is major abdominal surgery and you will receive detailed advice from the hospital about what you should and should not do to promote healing and recovery. This is not the time to prove you are superwoman, however much your adrenaline-fuelled euphoria or your deep belief that giving birth is not a medical event makes you want to get up and on with life at full throttle. Please, just pause for a moment and consider the fact that the physical and emotional demands of looking after a young baby are going to continue for months into the future. Your sleep will be broken for months… you won't be able to sleep 12 hours to set things straight if you take on too much and feel like you are about to collapse physically or emotionally. Set a sensible precedent – look after yourself from the start and it will be so much easier and more pleasurable to look after your baby.

Planning your babymoon in advance and telling friends and family about it is a way to ensure that you have the time and space to transition from pregnant woman to mother. If your partner is able to be home, taking the time to simply hang out together and relax and get to know your baby will help establish your sense of family. Hormones are in a state of flux: oxytocin, that wonderful love hormone, is flowing free, as is prolactin to establish breastfeeding. Levels of oestrogen and progesterone are rebalancing over the next few days and weeks, and having loved ones around you to simply hold you and be with you will help you at those times when you feel down or anxious. The emotional somersaults you experience make you vulnerable and open, and responsive to your little one: they make it easier to snuggle and be close to your baby. To simply be there, drinking them into your system. The hormones may also make you feel sad, confused and overwhelmed – just like your baby at times – so you are more able to empathise with their experience. Your feelings will settle down, just as your baby will: you just need time and loving support. Sharing your feelings is important, as is accepting them and not feeling guilty if it isn't all positive or if your feeling is one of numbness for a while. You have been through a rite of passage and you need time to process that. The 'Being inside' relaxation on page 32 can be helpful at times when you are feeling emotionally overwhelmed or as a daily practice. It is particularly soothing when you are unable to sleep but too tired to do much of anything else.

Think of your babymoon as an investment in your

future as a family. It's your opportunity to really get to know your baby and how she shows you what she needs, to help her feel safe and to help yourself get used to living without a schedule or to-do list. It makes total sense that you also follow the rhythm your baby sets you, sleeping when she sleeps, and eating frequent, regular nutritious meals and snacks. Think of it as living on 'baby time' and keep in mind that it is a temporary arrangement. As you notice what your baby's tendencies are, you can support them by ensuring the right environment for her at those general times of day. For example, if your baby seems wide awake at 8am and then tired at around 10–11am, don't invite visitors for 10am to get her too excited to rest. If your baby finds it easiest to sleep when she is either in the sling or a pram, then help her get a good nap by doing just that when she seems tired. Think of it as underlining the rhythm she needs.

It will take a while for your baby to show you how adaptable she is to change, but by about three months of age you will probably know whether your baby seems to embrace variety or if she is disturbed by it. One baby will simply sleep when she needs to, taking many short naps during the day, while another will regularly sleep, for example, from 10–11am and 2–3pm, but might need to be in a particular place to do so. Both these situations have advantages: baby one is more flexible to your needs, but not predictable, so planning can be trickier, and while baby two makes different demands of you, she is predictable but not flexible. And of course the third option is predictable and flexible... it does exist, but we are not all lucky enough to have babies like that!

Your newborn baby is used to simply doing what she needs to. She will be hungry whenever her tummy is empty, which given that it starts off the size of a cherry and grows rapidly in the first two weeks to the size of a large egg, doesn't stay the same for long. Poo production in the first few weeks is usually little and often and linked to her feeding: food goes in and poo comes out, sometimes at the same time. This will also change over time and if you are breastfeeding your baby she may poo less frequently. Once she reaches about eight weeks the frequency of her poo will change and can be anything from a couple of times a day to once every week or two (there is little waste left over from breastmilk). A bottle-fed baby will likely poo on a daily basis and is more prone to constipation because of the nature of formula. Sleeping, cuddling and playing vary even more between individuals. Each baby is so different: some sleep almost all the time, and some seem to sleep hardly at all, but most babies prefer to be close to their parents, either held or sleeping on them. Some individuals are better able to settle alone. As far as your baby is concerned, as long as her needs are met she will be happy, so the quicker you find out how to do that the easier your life will be.

What about you?

After a few weeks of simply 'hanging out' and doing what your baby wants, you may start to wonder when it will all end. When will you be able to get the sleep/

food/break you really need? When will you be able to start to follow your own interests again, and have those interests changed? For many women, becoming a mother is a precursor to massive changes in priorities, expectations and even values. The hormonal rebalancing act that your body does after you give birth, those 'third-day baby blues' that you hear about, will take you to extremes, from feeling intensely loved-up, mellow and motherly to completely numb, miserable, terrified or even angry. Once the hormones settle many women go into 'survival mode' as the weeks pass and the torture of waking up every hour or two to feed your baby starts to hit. You really don't have the energy to start questioning your life choices. It is enough to manage to get up and get through the day (notice I didn't even say get dressed or washed). As you near the end of the second month, as your baby starts to smile with more intention and feed less often and things get easier to manage, don't be surprised if your emotions rise to the surface again. I observe this happening to many new mums, and it can be very disconcerting for them. Just as things seem more manageable practically speaking, the psychological side of this whole venture starts to get a bit more tricky. Of course the issues are varied. Some women feel they have lost their identity, others have found one, many start to feel isolated and alone, some of us are worried about going back to work, others long to be able to focus on their work again. Happy, sad, impatient or thoughtful, moving between emotions is normal, but getting stuck in one or other of them is something you want to avoid.

Interesting, isn't it, that this is the very thing you are teaching your child... emotional regulation. It seems it is a challenge for everyone concerned in this family venture.

If you have been pregnant then hopefully the process of the pregnancy has helped you become aware of your emotional resources, and perhaps created new ones. Breath work and the restorative poses that you did in the yoga class, the hypnobirthing course visualisations, the 'going for a walk every day' or taking an afternoon nap. All these various ways you looked after yourself and your baby in preparation for the birth can go on serving you once the baby is here. For partners or parents who were not pregnant themselves it is also well worth taking a moment to recognise what you habitually do to help yourself calm down, cheer up and feel contented. Once you are aware of what your resources are you can get creative in finding ways of making sure they are there for you now, when you need them. Take a moment to go through the checklist below to help you clarify what is important to you, then you can work out what is actually possible for you in the present situation.

Emotional resource checklist

What usually helps you feel better when you feel stressed or overwhelmed?

- I need to be physically active. I usually do that

by _____

- I need to be alone for a while and _____
- I unwind by being in nature or near water. I can do that by _____
- I like to lose myself in narrative (book/film/series) so I will _____
- Company helps me process feelings. I can talk, laugh, and share with _____
- Listening to music, playing an instrument or singing helps me, particularly _____
- I like to eat or drink nice things, like _____
- Sleep helps. I just need to rest. I can get extra sleep by _____
- I find meditative practice/breathwork/yoga helpful, so I can _____
- I like therapeutic touch, like massage/shiatsu, so I will book.....

The basics of your days

Now that you have identified what worked for you pre-baby, let's get some realistic expectations on the table and work out how you can most easily use your favourite resources once baby is here.

Physical release

It is great to be active again after the birth, but you do need to know what you are doing and you will need to rest for some time. If you had a c-section then you need to let your body recover after what is major abdominal surgery, and even if you had a vaginal birth you will need a few weeks' recovery time. So what can you do? First off, find out where your local postnatal exercise class is and find out how to book a place. You can usually join six weeks after a vaginal birth and 10–12 weeks after a caesarean, but many new mums don't feel ready to exercise quite so soon. Be kind to yourself, but make sure you do it. Your body has spent nine months changing alignment, and relaxin levels in your body remain high for some months, destabilising joints and affecting your balance and your pelvic floor. Specialist instruction is really important and will get your posture, pelvic floor and abdominal muscles to a point where you can go on to take regular exercise classes safely.

You don't have to wait for a class to move your body though. Taking time to roll around on your bed or your floor, doing gentle stretches and those basic pelvic floor exercises (Kegels) where you breathe out as you tighten the muscles round your vagina and anus and breathe in as you release them. These are safe to start as soon as you can after a vaginal delivery as the movement helps bring blood to the perineal area for healing. If you have had a tear or episiotomy, do ask your midwife or doctor for advice. Any low-impact exercise is good postnatally: dancing around to your favourite music, or rolling on the floor as your baby lies next to you enjoying stretching and resting… just think little and often rather than 'It's my hour of exercise'. Little three-minute blocks throughout the day soon add up. You may find that your baby really enjoys sharing your physical activity, so a walk with the pram or babywearing is an important part of every day once your babymoon is over.

Eating

One of the benefits of breastfeeding is that you need to up your calorie intake considerably: you need around 300–500 extra calories, or a small extra meal. The tricky thing is making sure those calories give you good nutrition and not just sugar or fat (the two types of food we tend to turn to when tired or stressed). Buy in the healthy stuff that is easy to pick at if you are too occupied to make yourself a proper meal and let your visitors supply you with goodies and treats (or even better, a home-cooked meal). Eating is a pretty popular way of responding to stress. The first few months of raising a baby are stressful enough without putting yourself under diet or guilt pressure. Do what you feel comfortable with, just make sure you get good nutrition.

Distraction

Books, movies, radio – something to occupy your mind can be crucial for some of us. You may be surprised that you can't concentrate very well at first, so it's probably not the time to listen to an audio version of *Ulysses* by James Joyce, but audio books, podcasts and radio keep many of us going through the darkest times. Screens can be a bit more problematic when we have so many of them in our lives. Your baby needs your attention, and you need to be so aware of the tiny signs that they make to indicate their moods, needs and desires, so watching a screen instead of your baby can get in the way of important bonding and learning processes. Having said that, sleeping babies do not see what you are doing. Remember though – you need to sleep too and we all know how mesmerising watching a screen can be. Sleeping when your baby sleeps is the only way to get through the early weeks unless you have the money to pay for a maternity nurse, so use screens with care!

Company

It can be surprisingly lonely and isolating to look after a young baby and having friends and family to support you is important, particularly if your relationships are an important resource for you. At first many people find the prospect of leaving the house with the baby daunting, so make sure that people are ready to come over and keep you company if needed. Try to connect with local people who you meet at antenatal activities before your baby is here and support each other with a call or a visit when needed. Even if your family is around you to help it can be so nice to share your experiences with someone to whom it is all equally new.

Space and time to yourself

Whether you need to sit in the bath, nap or play your instrument alone, time and space for yourself can be the hardest things to achieve. Not only do you have a baby who, certainly for the first few weeks, has unpredictable hunger or may well decide that being in your arms is the only comfortable place in the world, but you may also have internal pressures that might make you ambivalent about leaving your baby in someone else's arms (even those of another parent). So even when you know you need alone time, you may find it hard to motivate yourself to seek it. The problem is that your need does not just vanish, so finding a way to fulfil it while parenting a young baby is important. The key here is your attitude and your expectations. A day at the spa may be what you would like, but if you manage a 20-minute soak in the bath with candles while someone takes the baby out for a walk round the block, and you treat it as a special time just to relax and enjoy... that is probably manageable. And if you ensure that this is a set ritual, and that your partner/mother/baby sitter or best friend is scheduled in each week, it will give you something to look forward to at times of stress. In the groups I run we practise ways of taking just a moment to focus in on ourselves: three deep breaths, feeling your body relax, or sitting down and simply listening to a favourite piece of music without making to-do lists in your head, or writing one page of your journal every day. Simple mindfulness techniques can make your feel less overwhelmed and maintain your emotional resilience.

If you are finding things hard, communicate with your partner, friends and/or professionals to get you through the rough patches. Your needs are as important as your baby's – how you feel forms the primary environment for your baby's emotional development. It is no luxury to take time to look after yourself. It is simply sensible, good parenting. And it isn't just mothers who can feel emotionally vulnerable or overwhelmed. There is more to paternity leave than the practicalities of living with a baby, so make sure you take time to simply talk, share and be together. Be as kind to yourselves as you are to your little one.

SOME FINAL WORDS

So this is where I leave you. I hope that this book has helped you gain a deeper understanding of your baby's needs. I hope the explorations have extended your awareness and that you feel more resourced in this journey of discovery that is parenthood. The discovery I speak about is as much about ourselves as our children. Along the way you will surprise yourself with your resourcefulness and also your ineptitude, experience soaring joy and the depths of despair, feel at one with every other parent in the world and sometimes so very alone in your particular situation. However much you strive for some kind of perfection, you are human, and it just doesn't come with the territory. Love your baby the best you can, respect their needs and try to meet them. Sometimes you will succeed, sometimes you will fail –

and the fails will teach you the most. So welcome them and learn from them and know that you will find your rhythm together, then they will change and you will find another one, and so it goes on!

In this age of global connection and distant family, make sure you build a community of support around you. Use the internet as well as your local community to reach out when you feel lonely or bored. Don't ever feel afraid of asking for help or support: we never stop learning through relationships. You will find fellow parents with a similar outlook to your own, and be amazed at people's kindness and generosity. Enjoy it and pay it forward when you get the chance.

And finally, while you are busy learning about your little one you will also have the opportunity to learn about yourself. Let your baby inspire you as you watch how keenly they follow their interests, how freely they share their love and joy, how fiercely they demand kindness, cuddles and connection. Join them in exploring the world around you with fresh eyes and an open heart. Let their excitement at being alive spark your own creative soul and send it out into the world to inspire others.

APPENDIX:
WHEN THINGS ARE
UNUSUALLY DIFFICULT

In Chapter 5 we took a look at the nitty-gritty reality of your first three months with your baby and how you can bolster your resilience in simple and practical ways to ensure that this first trimester is a big fluffy dream of joy. Hopefully all that we have discussed so far has helped you to better understand both your newborn baby and yourself as a mother, and given you some ideas about how to navigate the early days of parenthood and build lasting bonds with your baby. But what if your situation is especially difficult, and you fear that something is 'wrong' with you or your baby? One possibility is that unresolved trauma is having an effect. Trauma is a frightening word, especially when applied to your newborn baby. And yet if your baby is behaving in a way that alarms you:

either they are incredibly sensitive and quick to cry, or perhaps they are the direct opposite – sleepy, quiet and withdrawn, completely in their 'inner world' – or if you had a difficult birth that has left you feeling anxious, angry or numb and depressed, you may well be suffering from trauma and some understanding of what trauma is, how it affects us and how you can address it will help you.

This is not an easy subject to write about for new parents, and the simple fact that anxiety plays such a big role in the first few months of parenting makes many professionals unwilling to mention trauma for fear of planting this particular seed of worry in people's minds. It is a delicate thing, new parenthood, and sometimes it is important to focus on building up your ability to stay calm rather than adding yet another reason to be worried and stressed. Birth, for most women and their babies, involves some level of stress, and if you start off looking for signs of trauma, you will invariably find them. The behaviour I described above: sensitive or sleepy baby, anxious or feeling down mother, is *normal for a few weeks*, until parents find their rhythm, hormones settle and babies acclimatise to the world. When it persists, or if you feel yourself getting stuck in a difficult place emotionally, it is important to address the problem.

Too often I work with families who have an extremely difficult life for months and months, putting it down to their baby's particularly sensitive personality, because they are unaware that the behaviour could be the result of a traumatic perinatal (before or after the birth) experience.

When we address trauma promptly it is easier to deal with and we avoid the spiral of misunderstanding that can so easily arise when parents feel pressure to try and change their baby's behaviour without understanding the reason for it, or indeed when parents are unable to respond to their baby's needs due to their own trauma.

We know that trauma is not something babies just 'grow out of'. It can have long-term physical and psychological effects, impacting behaviour, learning skills and the ability to form relationships throughout our lives. Birth trauma from the parents' perspective is linked to postnatal depression. A systemic review of studies looking at the link between birth experience and postnatal depression, published in the *Midwifery* journal in August 2016, concluded that 'the weight of evidence suggests that a negative birth experience may contribute to postnatal depression.'[1] So let's get on with exploring trauma, and we will start with some definitions.

What is trauma?

The word trauma is often used to describe an event, but in actual fact it refers to our *experience*: not what has happened, but how what has happened has affected us. This is an important distinction, because it means that the same event can be perceived in different ways by different people. While a life-threatening event is more likely to be traumatising than, say, the experience of having a blood test, trauma is subjective. You can't assume that just because the birth was difficult for you, your baby will be traumatised by it. It also works the other way: a birth experience that you are happy with may nonetheless have been traumatic for your baby. Trauma is also used to describe a physical injury: thus, bruising or grazing of the perineum during birth would be described as trauma to the perineal tissue, and so would a tear or a prolapse. A baby might also be physically injured during the birth process, and this can range from relatively minor issues such as bruising to fracture of the collarbone, which a recent study showed to be the most common birth injury at 0.41% of total live births.[2] (Just to reassure you, if you are reading this prior to giving birth – in all the cases studied these fractures healed and caused no lasting damage).

For example, a baby who has difficulty turning their head to one side due to birth injury has an obvious physical problem, but it is one which might also be affecting the ability of the nervous system to move from activation to calm due to a compression of the cranial nerves that support the calming branches of our nervous system (the parasympathetic). This might make them anxious and difficult to settle. If left unaddressed, it might make you think of your baby as particularly sensitive, perhaps even difficult to live with. In this way their restriction may become their 'personality' in your eyes, and even if the condition eases during the normal process of physical development and their head is freer, the physical and neurological patterns that have been established or the compensations they have made in order to bypass them may persist. I hope it is now rare for paediatricians not to take issues of alignment and physical restriction/ injury during the birth process seriously and refer babies for treatment promptly. Professionals who can treat this kind of issue include physiotherapists, osteopaths, cranio-sacral therapists and chiropractors, obviously all with specific training and experience of working with babies. Your doctor, midwife or health visitor should be able to refer you to specialists in your area and it is always worthwhile connecting with local parents' groups for personal recommendations.

Physical trauma may be obvious, but what about when there is no visible problem? What do we mean by trauma in this case? Trauma describes a response to an event, rather than the event itself, as we've already discussed. Trauma is what happens when an event completely overwhelms our nervous system and in so doing floods it with stress hormones, activating our fight, flight or freeze responses. Trauma can be the result of a single event, like a forceps delivery, a surgical procedure or even induction methods that prompt immediate, strong contractions. Trauma can also be created by something more sustained, for example a toxic atmosphere in the womb caused by drugs or alcohol, a parent who consistently disregards a baby's needs, or a parent who is unpredictable and inconsistent in their responses, perhaps as a result of having had a difficult childhood themselves.

If you are feeling worried simply reading this, please don't be. Feel your feet on the ground for a moment, relax your shoulders and remember that our nervous system is designed to deal with traumatic events. Problems arise when trauma is not processed and released but remains within your nervous system. Prioritising your baby's sense of safety, preventing overstimulation, giving them time and space to express feelings, in fact all the handling tips that you have read about so far, as well as the information in Chapter 2, will go a long way to helping your baby with any trauma they may have experienced and could well be enough to help them recover their equilibrium.

So what is actually happening physically when we experience trauma? When we feel threatened our nervous system kicks into action and gets our body ready to respond in one of three ways: fight, flee or freeze. The first two responses activate our sympathetic nervous system by releasing adrenaline and noradrenaline, which produce a surge of energy: raising our heart rate, speeding up our breathing and preparing muscles to either run away or do battle. The third response, which kicks in when it becomes apparent that fleeing and fighting are not possible, activates the dorsal vagus nerve and puts us in a 'frozen' or withdrawn, disassociated state of mind. Infants are most susceptible to entering this state, since they are incapable of either running away or fighting. While on the surface this frozen state may seem like calm, all the energy released by the adrenaline rush of fear is still there underneath the silent surface, and it needs to be discharged or it will start to affect your baby's ability to respond and engage with the world around them.

These reactions date back to our mammalian ancestors, and are perhaps easiest to describe using the example of an antelope being chased by a lioness. At the first sign of the threat our antelope will run away. If the lioness catches up, it might try and fight back with its horns, but when this fails the only option the antelope has is to go limp, into an unconscious state, which at worst means it won't feel the pain of death, or at best, may prompt the lioness to decide it must be ill or unsafe to eat and lose interest in her meal. Let's take the best-case scenario: the lioness goes away, leaving our antelope alive. After some time the antelope will stand up, start to tremble, pant and breathe deeply and run away, discharging the energy from that initial sympathetic system charge. The nervous system is once more in balance.

If we have a baby in our arms, not an antelope, how do we know she has experienced trauma? This is where it can get tricky. Sometimes it is likely that there will some degree of trauma to deal with. Being separated from close contact with her parents after birth, for example, is a stressor for your baby, and whether it is due to illness, prematurity or something else, you should be encouraged to spend as much time in skin-to-skin contact with your baby as possible to alleviate their internal distress once you can. But if there is no obvious event to consider, all you might have to go on is gut feeling and your baby's behaviour.

Perhaps you have a baby who is unsettled, uncomfortable, startles easily, naps seldom and sleeps badly. You might notice that your baby has a relatively tense body, or seems to dislike being held close and cuddled. People may remark on her good head control, but fail to see that she is bracing her shoulders and neck in tension and her neck is stiff and inflexible, not balanced and supported. Your baby might want to suckle for long periods of time without actually feeding (it is a baby's way to release spinal tension, as well as claim their connection with you). Other babies may have tipped over into the freeze response: they may be very sleepy and hard to engage with when awake. The 'inner focus' that I described earlier may be their default behaviour rather than something they do from time to time.

Most of these 'indicators of trauma' are also simply the way a baby will behave when they are born: after all, we all need to process stress and effort, and things should become calmer and more relaxed, or in the case of a sleepy baby, more alert, over the first few weeks. But some babies don't seem to adjust and in these cases you may want to consult someone for extra support. Depending on where you live you may have access to health visitors that are sympathetic and can offer referrals to perinatal psychology services, or you might be interested in working with a specialist cranio-sacral, somatic or perinatal therapist. There are different ways of working with trauma and practitioners will use their particular approach to help the baby discharge the adrenaline rush that is still in their system and help them feel safe and secure again. This will often involve working with parents to respond more appropriately to the cues their baby is giving them, or process any trauma they themselves may have experienced. Hands-on therapeutic techniques might also be used to support your baby. For more information on this topic see the list of further reading at the back of the book.

It is well established in the medical field that trauma is a condition that can affect both parents and babies. If you are the one who feels traumatised, it can be particularly hard to help your baby regain their equilibrium. You may feel unable to regulate your own distress and anxiety, or you may have entered a numb, cut-off sense of self (that freeze again), which makes it hard to respond to your child with your full attention. While you may be going through the motions and seeing to your child's needs perfectly satisfactorily, if you feel like you are only half present, if you find it hard to play or engage with your child, or you find yourself constantly distracted, you need to seek some help and support. The quality of your relationship with your child, your ability to respond sensitively and consistently to their needs, is what creates the quality of their attachment to you.

It is important to be aware of what trauma is, how it may manifest and address it if you feel that you are affected by it. I don't want you to lose sight of the fact that sensitive, responsive parenting – that natural impulse we have to soothe, comfort and hold our babies close to our hearts – is designed to ameliorate the shock of the birth process.

The last 50 years has seen an explosion of interest and research in neurological development. Technological advances have enabled us to watch a live human brain respond to stimulus as well as discern increasingly smaller structures within it. Interdisciplinary research by neuroscientists, psychologists, immunologists, biochemists and philosophers is exploring the integrated way our mind and body cooperate and the physical systems which enable this. Neuroscientific research has brought additional insights into the importance of emotional regulation as a skill that is both possessed and acquired.

The nervous system operates not only as an electrical circuit, but also on a biochemical basis. In the 1970s and 1980s we started to research how peptides (such as endorphins) affect our brains, and researchers like Dr Candace Pert[3] discovered that our brains are intrinsically emotional. The emotions we feel not only produce physical responses that are visible, such as blushing when you feel embarrassed, but they also affect our whole bodies because they effect changes to our actual cells. Our brain is not like a computer, an empty hard drive waiting for its software. We humans are way more complex. For a start our brain is just part of the central nervous system that extends throughout our body. This system functions together with our whole organism, experiences interact with emotions, emotions interact with hormones, hormones interact with organs, blood circulation, our senses and our movements: we are constantly adjusting and responding to our environment as a whole being. Following the birth of your child these hormones help you feel with an intensity that is more closely matched to your baby's experience, helping you relate to the drama that is going on for them. The emotional somersaults you experience make you vulnerable and open, responsive to your little one; they make it easier to snuggle and be close to your baby. To simply be there, drinking them into your system. The hormones may also make you feel sad, confused, overwhelmed – just like your baby at times! – so you are more able to empathise with their experience.

So rather than look at the brain in isolation I want to back up a step and consider something more fundamental that affects our brain, and our body's abilities and its function. It is our feeling of safety, that place where we are content and open to learning. The 'set point' which Sue Gerhardt refers to is a physical thing and it is also a state of mind. The state of arousal that is described is an emotional one, and learning to regulate our emotions starts within our mother's womb and continues through baby and childhood often past adolescence into our adult years. It is important to underline just how much we rely on our caregivers to help us learn how to regulate our emotions, and why it is worthwhile for parents to focus on this particular aspect of their baby's care from the very start. Put simply, we thrive when we feel safe, calm and attentive.

So, if you are struggling, the less you fight your feelings the easier it will be to ride them out. Sharing them is important, as is accepting them and not feeling guilty if parenthood isn't all positive or if your feeling is one of numbness for a while. You have been through a rite of passage and you need time to process that. The 'Being inside' relaxation on page 32 can be helpful at times when you are feeling emotionally overwhelmed or as a daily practice, and is particularly soothing when you are unable to sleep but too tired to do much of anything else. And while you figure out what you want to do, soothe your baby, protect her 'being inside time', take things slow, curl her up close to you when she needs support and reassure her of her safety.

Our understanding of trauma and the way it can influence our lives if left unaddressed has deepened considerably in recent years, but this knowledge may not be at the fingertips of every professional you encounter, so I think it is important to have some insight into how trauma works, what you can do to help yourself and your baby and who you can turn to if you need more support. It is important to remember that trauma is a survival response to an event that is overwhelming to us: it is the way our nervous system protects us and allows us to keep going.

The calmer you can be as parents, the more it will help your baby recover from the normal stress of the birth. However, recent years have seen a great deepening of our knowledge about perinatal and birth trauma, and you may well find yourself on the internet, becoming more and more concerned as you read about the potential effects of trauma. Trauma is quite a buzz word at the moment and if your birth experience was negative and traumatic, being told that 'all's well that ends well' or 'all that matters is a healthy baby' is simply not good enough and will not help you regain your equilibrium. Your midwife and doctor will be aware that processing the experience, perhaps by working through it with a specialist therapist or counsellor, is far more beneficial in the long run than trying to sweep your feelings under the carpet and focus entirely on your baby. Professional help is not an over-reaction. It is an investment in your future as a family and there are a number of therapies that can be helpful. Osteopathy and chiropractic therapy have become popular in recent years and can be very supportive, both in correcting any physical misalignments, and in helping you and your baby release tension and recover. Midwives, perinatal psychologists, counsellors and somatic therapists may also be specialists in this field of work. Speaking to close friends and family members may also be helpful, but their emotional involvement may make it hard for you to be honest about your feelings, especially if you feel negative towards your baby. If you feel you need more support, don't be afraid to seek it. Trauma and postnatal depression are best addressed as fast as possible for your whole family's benefit: your doctor can refer you for counselling, or you may be able to access maternity mental health support or see a counsellor of your choice privately. Your baby was part of the experience that you are dealing with and she will benefit if you can process and come to terms with what happened. Postnatal depression in fathers is also now increasingly recognised and understood, and fathers who are struggling should also seek support.

I hope that this discussion of trauma as it relates to you and your baby has not freaked you out. My intention is not to frighten or worry you: if either of you need help to process your experiences, there is no shame in that – you haven't failed. In seeking support, you are demonstrating the very qualities of responsiveness and care that have been our focus in this book. The whole giving birth and looking after a baby experience is a big, emotional, messy and wonderful thing. It can feel like the best and the worst decision you ever made in your life – at the same time! Please remember that change is the name of the game: you are changing and so is your baby, and any situation you find yourself in will inevitably pass. Let this reassure you in times that are more difficult.

ACKNOWLEDGEMENTS

This book grew out of Ania's practice as a somatic movement educator working with parents and babies over many years in Manchester and Berlin. Although too numerous to mention individually, we would like to acknowledge how central those interactions were to her work, and ultimately to the knowledge she shares in this book.

It would seem wrong to not mention Ania's teacher, Linda Hartley, and the community of IBMT somatic practitioners who formed the bedrock of her professional circle. Deserving of particular mention are Kerstin Wellhofer and Beverley Nolan with whom Ania collaborated closely, sharing ideas and perspectives, and who provided invaluable help with proofing the text and suggesting amendments. We would like to thank her colleagues from Diversity and Balance, Berlin – Heike Kuhlmann, Ka Rustler and Adalisa Menghini – with whom she taught and who further contributed to the production of the book itself. And finally we would extend our thanks to Catherine Rees, who provided such excellent voice recordings for the somatic explorations which are featured in this book.

REFERENCES

Introduction

1. Attachment theory is a psychological model developed by British psychologist, psychiatrist and psychoanalyst John Bowlby (1907-1991). en.wikipedia.org/wiki/Attachment_theory

Chapter 1

1. Sue Gerhardt *Why Love Matters: how affection shapes a baby's brain* p18
2. Alva Noë *Out of Our Heads: Why you are not your brain and other lessons from the Biology of Consciousness* p65
3. Daniel N. Stern: *The Interpersonal world of the infant. A view from Psychoanalysis & Developmental Psychology* p46
4. Annie Brook *Birth's Hidden Legacy Vol 2. Treat Earliest origins of Shock and Attachment trauma in Adults, Children and Infants* p32
5. Lynne Murray and Liz Andrews *The Social Baby – Understanding Babies' Communication from Birth* p27
6. Lynne Murray *The Psychology of Babies: How relationships support development from birth to two* p11
7. Kirsten Weir: 'The Girl Who Smelled Pink' *Nautilus* nautil.us/issue/26/color/the-girl-who-smelled-pink
8. Daniel N. Stern: *The Interpersonal world of the infant. A view from Psychoanalysis & Developmental Psychology* p50–52
9. Google Scholar: Uvnäs-Moberg, K., Widstrom, A.M., Marchini, G. and Winberg, J. (1987). 'Release of GI hormones in mother and infant by sensory stimulation'. *Acta Paediatr. Scand.* 76, 851–860. doi: 10.1111/j.1651-2227.1987.tb17254.x
10. www.babycenter.com/0_pacifiers-pros-cons-and-smart-ways-to-use-them_128.bc

Chapter 2

1. Deane Juhan *Job's Body*, p35
2. *The Moving Child: How movement matters in a child's wellbeing.* (2017) dir. Hana Kamea Kemble. themovingchild.com
3. David Linden, 'The Science of Touching and Feeling' TEDxUNC, www.youtube.com/watch?v=lW8pJ7E9taQ
4. 'Neonatal Anesthesia – The Origins of Controversy'. Essay for the Osler Student Essay Contest written by Sunny Wei, mentored by Dr Thomas Schlich, www.mcgill.ca/library/files/library/wei_sunny_2016.pdf www.nocirc.org/symposia/second/chamberlain.html. University of Oxford News 21.4.2015, www.ox.ac.uk/news/2015-04-21-babies-feel-pain-adults
5. *Can Fam Physician.* 1989 May; 35: 1049–1054. 'Pain Perception in the Neonate'. Deana K. Midmer, www.ncbi.nlm.nih.gov/pmc/articles/PMC2280358/
6. 'The importance of touch in development' Evan L. Ardiel, MSc and Catharine H. Rankin, PhD. 2010. www.ncbi.nlm.nih.gov/pmc/articles/PMC2865952/#b1-pch15153

Chapter 4

1. Emmi Pikler *Se mouvoir en liberté dès le premier âge*, Paris, P.U.F, 1979
2. Dewey, C.; Fleming, P.; Golding, J.; The Alspac Study Team (1998). 'Does the Supine Sleeping Position Have Any Adverse Effects on the Child? II. Development in the First 18 Months'. *Pediatrics.* 101 (1): e5. doi:10.1542/peds.101.1.e5. PMID 9417169.
3. www.aap.org/en-us/about-the-aap/aap-press-room/Pages/American-Academy-of-Pediatrics-Announces-New-Recommendations-for-Childrens-Media-Use.aspx

Appendix

1. 'The birth experience and women's postnatal depression: A systematic review' Aleeca F. Bell PhD, RN, CNM(Assistant Professor) and Ewa Andersson PhD, RNM (Senior Lecturer), https://doi.org/10.1016/j.midw.2016.04.014

2. *Pediatr Int.* 2015;57(1):60-3. doi: 10.1111/ped.12497. Epub 2014 Nov 25. 'Neonatal clavicular fracture: recent 10 year study', Ahn, E.S., Jung, M.S., Lee, Y.K., Ko, S.Y., Shin, S.M., Hahn, M.H. www.ncbi.nlm.nih.gov/pubmed/25203556

3. Dr Candace Pert, *Molecules of Emotion: Why You Feel the Way You Feel*, Simon & Schuster, 1999.

FURTHER READING AND RESOURCES

Sue Gerhardt, *Why Love Matters: How Affection Shapes A Baby's Brain*, Routledge, 2014

Robin Grille, *Heart to Heart Parenting,* Vox Cordis Press, 2012

Gill Rapley and Tracey Murkett, *Baby-Led Breastfeeding,* Vermilion, 2012

Deborah Jackson *When Your Baby Cries*, Pinter & Martin, 2009

Naomi Stadlen, *What Mothers Do (Especially When It Looks Like Nothing)*, Piatkus, 2005

Lynne Murray and Liz Andrews, *The Social Baby: Understanding Babies' Communication From Birth*, CP Publishing, 2005

Daniel Stern, *Diary of a Baby: What Your Child Sees, Feels and Experiences*, Basic Books, 1992

Peter Levine and Maggie Kline, *Trauma through a Child's Eyes: Awakening the Ordinary Miracle of Healing*, North Atlantic Books, 2006

Bonnie Bainbridge Cohen, *Sensing, Feeling, and Action,* North Atlantic Books, 1993

Anat Baniel, *Kids Beyond Limits: The Anat Baniel Method for Awakening the Brain and Transforming the Life of Your Child with Special Needs,* Tarcher Perigee, 2012

Annie Brook, *Birth's Hidden Legacy (How Surprising Beliefs From Infancy Limit Successful Child and Adult Behavior, Volume 1)* and *Birth's Hidden Legacy (Treat Earliest*

*Origins of Shock and Attachment Trauma in Adults,
Children, and Infants, Volume 2).*

Emmi Pikler *Give me time. The independent movement of
the child's development to go free. Findings, articles and
lectures,* with Anna Tardos, Pflaum, München 2001/3

*Peaceful baby – happy mother. Pedagogical advice of a
pediatrician,* Herder, Freiburg 2008/9

Se mouvoir en liberté dès le premier âge, Paris, P.U.F, 1979

Breastfeeding support

UK National Breastfeeding Helpline: 0300 100 0212
Run by the Breastfeeding Network (BfN) and the
Association of Breastfeeding Mothers (ABM).
www.nationalbreastfeedinghelpline.org.uk

UK Breastfeeding Network: 0300 100 0210
Lines are open 9.30am–9.30pm every day and live
webchat service.
www.breastfeedingnetwork.org.uk/chat

La Leche League UK helpline
For a list of local supporters see *www.laleche.org.uk/call*

NCT helpline: 0300 330 0700
Practical and emotional support in feeding your baby.
www.nct.org.uk/parenting/about-breastfeeding

UK Drugs in Breastmilk helpline
For queries about the safety of medications and
breastmilk. *www.breastfeedingnetwork.org.uk/detailed-
information/drugs-in-breastmilk*

Australia:
Australian Breastfeeding Association
 www.breastfeeding.asn.au/breastfeeding-helpline

Canada:
La Leche League Canada www.lllc.ca

New Zealand:
La Leche League NZ lalecheleague.org.nz/get-help

United States:
La Leche League USA www.lllusa.org
Infant Risk Centre (medications) *www.infantrisk.com*

INDEX

Also from Pinter & Martin

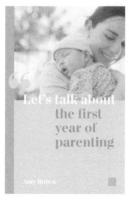

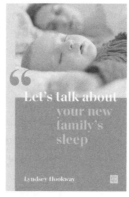

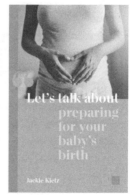

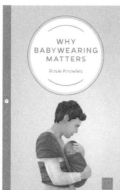

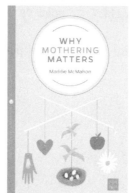

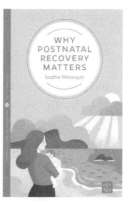

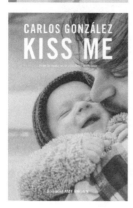

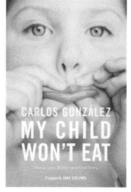

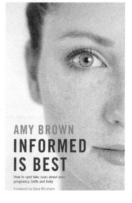